Is it **IBS** or Your

DIET?

**A Unique, Pivotal, and "Out of the Box"
Book about Irritable Bowel Syndrome**

Is it **IBS** or Your
DIET?

A Unique, Pivotal, and "Out of the Box" Book about Irritable Bowel Syndrome

M. Farivar, MD

Published by Best Seller Publishing®, St. Augustine, FL
Best Seller Publishing® is a registered trademark.
Printed in the United States of America.
ISBN: 978-1-959840-06-0

For more information, please write:
Best Seller Publishing®
53 Marine Street
St. Augustine, FL 32084
or call 1 (626) 765-9750
Visit us online at: www.BestSellerPublishing.org

Thanks to Mr. Soheil Givi
for his invaluable assistance
with initial formatting.

CONTENTS

PREFACE

Millions of people are suffering from IBS symptoms in the United States. From those only 25% seek medical attention, and in 5% (a tip of the iceberg) symptoms are severe enough that they'll be referred to a gastroenterologist for further evaluation and treatment. Indeed about 30% of general G.I. referrals are IBS related.

IBS is the second most common cause of work related absenteeism and diminished work productivity after the common cold. Moreover, patients with IBS consume over 50% more healthcare resources than matched control without IBS.

Health related quality of life (HRQL) scores of IBS patients are similar to depression in mild to moderate cases, and class 3 congestive heart failure in more severe patients.

Briefly, IBS symptoms are bowel movements that occur more or less often than usual, stool that appears less solid and more watery or harder and lumpier than usual, and having bowel movements that changes abdominal discomfort. A feeling of urgency to have a bowel movement, feeling incomplete evacuation and the need to have to go again, passing mucus, bloating and excessive flatulence are other associated symptoms.

Most recent claims by experts about the pathophysiology of IBS are that diet, excess bile acids, intestinal microbiome dysbiosis and SIBO are responsible for the majority of IBS-D cases.

In a given patient Symptoms severity varies from day-to-day and does not have to be present daily or even weekly.

It is because of the high prevalence of IBS, and the fact that an educated public pays more attention to their health, especially in Western countries that a huge commercial market has been born. The American Gastroenterology Association (AGA)clinical practice guidelines press release and publications in May 2022 strongly recommends linaclotide for IBS constipation, and rifaximin for IBS diarrhea. (you may have seen commercials about the aforementioned medications on your TV).

The global IBS treatment market is estimated to be valued at 1,444.7 million US dollars in 2022 and to surpass 3902.2 million US dollars by 2030. Interested parties are planning workshops, infomercials, lectures, etc. to create awareness about IBS and promote targeted treatments. Soon we may see linaclotide 75mcg tablets and more being offered over the counter for IBS-C patients.

The IBS therapy field is already muddied and overwhelmed with slew of expensive probiotics, fiber supplements, peppermint oil, Gas-X, Lactaid products , Beano, gluten cutter, activated charcoal, multiple medications, alternative treatment like Yoga, acupuncture, psychotherapy, etc. all claiming to have a role in relieving IBS symptoms.

Commercial labs have not missed the opportunity to jump on the IBS band wagon, trying to reap the benefit when they can by charging desperate patients with intractable symptoms hundreds of dollars to test their blood for measuring antibodies (mostly IgG) to many different food peptides, hair analysis, stool tests for bacteria, candida, parasites, etc. to let these patient know what may be causing their symptoms. Needless to say the majority if not all of these treatments and tests are not approved by FDA and the GI scientific societies and offer no real and permanent solution.

Based on close to half a century practice as a board-certified gastroenterologist with academic appointments at Harvard and

Boston University medical schools, I believe that true IBS is exceedingly rare, and the majority of patients labeled as having IBS only have "normal" diet related symptoms, that may vary from one day to another, depending on their diet type and amount of offending food and drink consumed.

A smaller percentage of patients have easily identifiable and potentially important but treatable cause for their symptoms, but unfortunately have come under the "umbrella" of IBS.

In this book I have attempted to describe dietary factors that can cause IBS type symptoms, recommendations as how to recognize and modify them, and identify pitfalls in diagnosis of other diseases hiding under IBS umbrella.

A better informed consumer can help his/her health care provider identify other etiologies be it organic or functional, like dietary factors, intestinal microbiome dysbiosis, bile acid dysregulation, leaky gut, SIBO, food allergy, food sensitivity, etc. (see differential diagnosis).

The final chapter describes several interesting patients with "IBS" seen in my practice. They illustrate the importance of spending time for detailed daily dietary history, knowledge of pathophysiology of digestion and absorption, especially carbohydrates and their storage proteins, including: lactose, fructose, sucrose, fructans, galactans, (FODMAP), and not being satisfied when discovering one or even two etiologies in your patients.

WHAT IS IRRITABLE BOWEL SYNDROME (IBS)?

There are a wide spectrum of conditions, some serious and most not so serious, that can present with symptoms suggestive of IBS and are often misdiagnosed as IBS. In my experience, true IBS disease is extremely rare. IBS is described as a complex GI disorder of **unknown theology**, with clinical presentation of abdominal discomfort or **pain altering with bowel movements** (better or worse), and associated with **change in bowel habits (diarrhea or constipation). Symptoms needs not be daily or even weekly, as long as it occurs at least one day a week for three months of the last 12 months. It does not have to be consecutive days or month either.**

This is a very noncommittal description with moving parts, and unfair to those suffering from occasional "IBS" symptoms to be marked as having IBS disease.

It is postulated that IBS is a "multifactorial, polygenic, complex disorder affecting GI sensory and motor functions, causing different phenotypes of IBS (diarrhea, constipation or mixed)."

Because IBS is common, chronic, has no well-defined etiology, symptoms that could be daily, weekly or even monthly, it's advised and accepted by international GI societies, including the American

College of Gastroenterology, that diagnostic testing is not necessary if the patient meets Rome IV criteria for IBS.

"Physicians are advised to establish a positive diagnosis, and to reassure the patient that there's nothing seriously wrong (if Alarm symptoms are not present). They should ask them to focus on health and not illness, and set realistic goals for patients. Physicians should inform the patient that although this could be a lifelong problem, it may have more to do with their personality traits of being sensitive, anxious or uptight, in addition to possibly having issues related to psychosocial aspects of life at home, school, work, etc. The health care worker should try to manage the chief complaints with appropriate medications, while prescribing alternative treatment modalities such as psychotherapy, acupuncture, probiotics, and so on, in patients that are difficult to treat or satisfy."

This whole description of Rome criteria, pathophysiology and treatment often doesn't make sense.

It is believed that in the US, 15 to 20% of the population suffers from IBS, but only 25% of those affected by symptoms seek medical attention, and even a smaller percentage of them (a tip of the iceberg) are referred to a GI specialist. Indeed, with a combination of health care, illness behavior and psychiatric diagnoses, less than 5% of IBS patients consider their disease severe, even when experiencing constant symptoms. However, up to 40% of GI referrals from PCPs are for IBS. Furthermore, IBS patients constitute up to 30% of a given GI's practice, and accounts for 30% of health-related costs in gastroenterology.

IBS affects quality of life in ways similar to depression and, in severe cases, class three congestive heart failure. It is the second most common cause of work-related absenteeism after the common cold, and second to obesity in public health-related issues.

The reason that I decided to write this book is to guide those who are suffering about their "IBS" diagnosis and self-management. In my experience, educated IBS patients often visit Internet websites and look for information and advice first, followed by seeing a PCP, and eventually receiving a referral to a specialist as times goes on, only to be disappointed, because no matter where they try to seek advice, their answers are about the same (cookie cutter answers), with each giving incremental advice and information. The information can vary, depending on the level of interest and education on the subject on behalf of the patient or the websites. Factors ranging from changes in diet to an increase medications that can alter symptoms, procedures such as blood tests, stool tests, colonoscopies and upper Endoscopies (with or without biopsy) may provide clearer information. The end result more often than not is that frustrated patients will have to learn to live with IBS (setting up expectations). However, in recent years, again thanks to the abundance of information on the internet and from patients themselves, occasionally they'll discover the cause and proper treatment, and following it, they get better or their symptoms improve. IBS patients usually become a stable part of a GI practice, with frequent visits for years to come in order to renew their required prescriptions, in hopes of a "new miracle" to end their suffering.

"Advice usually starts with drink 8 to 10 glass of water daily, eat plenty of fruits and vegetables, take a cup of bran cereal or a tablespoon of psyllium powder (Metamucil) or a couple of tablespoons of raw bran daily." Other than drinking water—that is always good—everything else may make them feel worse. The PCP may also add an anti-spasmodic for pain, anti-diarrheal medication for diarrhea predominant IBS or laxatives for IBS-constipation. The GI Specialist may prescribe newer, more expensive medications with the same effect and if up to date a printed list of high-FODMAP foods to avoid. Since the diagnosis of IBS is symptom-based, depending on the knowledge base of the health care provider that the patient sees, the amount of tests performed can vary from none to several. I have seen a super-specialist professor, that goes by the Rome IV criteria for diagnosis of IBS (if the shoe fits wear it, that is the Rome IV criteria), perform minimal to no investigations and then recommend 7 G of fiber daily (a cup of high-fiber cereal daily like bran or Kashi), plus antispasmodic Dicyclomine for pain. However, in the same department, a different GI will get a set of blood and stool tests to check for gluten allergy and IBD

(Crohn's or colitis). Yet a third GI will order a colonoscopy and upper endoscopy to look for colitis, Crohn's, Celiac disease, etc. (Of course I don't agree with any of it.)

There is no specific test other than symptoms criteria for diagnosis of IBS, and treatment is guided towards relieving symptoms, such as abdominal discomfort, bloating, diarrhea, or constipation. Some patients with intractable symptoms are even referred for psychotherapy, acupuncture, and other forms of alternative therapy (CAM), including very expensive probiotics delivered weekly in dry ice. Because of the chronicity of symptoms of IBS, and the lack of definite therapy, patients are often not taken seriously. As a result, patients may end up doctor shopping in hopes of finding a "life-line", going from one specialist to another, often to no avail.

Unfortunately for IBS patients, this vicious cycle of frequent doctor visits, accompanied with the same complaint of "I'm not getting better," creates the image of a neurotic patient in the health care provider's mind. Even if the patient's symptoms are considered to be real, the provider may determine that the patient is just unhappy with the level of attention they are receiving, and that otherwise, there is nothing wrong with them. The patient has no signs of celiac or colitis. The provider simply changes the patient's meds and prescribes anxiolytics or antidepressants, then gives them another appointment for follow up.

IBS is not glorified, like Crohn's disease and Colitis, by doctors and drug companies. These patients, in terms of importance, are considered "the lowest man on the totem pole", and are often seen by nurse practitioners (NP) or physician assistants (PA). They are just numbers, used to fill the daily schedule of the office and supplement the establishment's income.

You may be surprised to know (I have seen it), that large healthcare systems and hospitals, as well as major teaching hospitals, don't take IBS patients seriously. Often, these institutions are not even equipped with the very basic and inexpensive instruments need in order to measure Hydrogen in exhaled breath. Without these instruments, they are unable to diagnose lactose, fructose and sucrose intolerance, nor the small intestinal bacterial overgrowth (SIBO) conditions that commonly contribute to the symptoms experienced by many IBS patients. They probably don't bother getting these instruments, either because they don't believe that these problems contribute to IBS symptoms, or insurance reimbursements for these tests are relatively low. They may say that they are too understaffed in the office or department to perform the breath tests. These tests can be done by an ordinary medical office worker with a minimal learning curve. While in private practice, I had three QuinTron breathalyzers for breath tests. Even on the Fridays that I was off, several patients could go to the office for their breath test. You'd be surprised to learn the numbers with positive results.

In my close to half a century of practice, I have seen many patients that are suffering from real IBS infrequently, as compared to patients with IBS symptoms that are related to one or more definable etiologies. Patients with real IBS are usually female, with severe chronic diarrhea and abdominal pain that respond to specific IBS meds. These patients often have cramps and mucus diarrhea during stressful situations. Others experience LLQ pain, tenderness and mucus diarrhea that colonoscopy reveals to be related to circular muscle hypertrophy and spasm, especially in the sigmoid colon region.

Other than some specific cause of IBS symptoms like Celiac and SIBO that will be discussed later, the major reason for "IBS" symptoms are most likely food related, and deserve more attention. The most common cause of these symptoms is the excessive use of High-FODMAP foods, or lactose and fructose intolerance.

The physiology of digestion and absorption is similar in all people. Humans have no enzymes to digest and absorb the FODMAP that is prominent in our healthy foods. These undigested, and therefore unabsorbed, food particles enter the large intestine to be digested(fermented) by colon bacteria, which produces, amongst other byproducts, "gas." However, the difference lies in the fact that people have varying dietary habits, whether from day to day, season to season, place to place, etc. The small or large amount of offending foods contained in a person's diet, in combination with limited storing capacity, challenges their tolerance level when it comes to gas, bloating, and changes in daily bowel habits. Large amounts of gas in a small frame, physically fit female will have difficulty expanding and may cause discomfort and bloating. Whereas a large amount of gas in a large male with huge colonic capacity with no shame of passing gas in public. Additionally, his intestinal walls can expand and accommodate extra gas and therefore reduce or not cause pain. Other factors like workplace environment, the availability of private bathrooms, allergies to foods, other medical problems like diabetes, and the frequency of eating out are among other contributors to symptoms. Also, it is known that people have different intestinal microbiome that deal with undigested food differently. Based on this fact, **every** individual eventually suffers more or less from IBS symptoms, it is only natural. IBS is considered a functional disorder and not organic. It is related to individual personality, environment, relationships between brain and gut, etc. The majority of people experiencing symptoms are normal, and those symptoms are related to diet. However, an individual's tolerance to these symptoms will vary, based on acceptance, sensitivity to health issues, level of education and degree of symptoms. Symptoms, if bothersome, can be managed by reducing or eliminating offending dietary items.

This book is designed to educate patients to self-eliminate the cause of IBS symptoms if possible, providing a step-by-step guidance to look for etiology.

GI centers, especially in busy hospitals and academic institutions, need to adopt uniform and universal IBS diagnosis and treatment protocols (certainly today's E&R is woefully inadequate). This change in attitude will help a large percentage of patients, previously diagnosed to have IBS, to be able to discard the medication they have been using daily (or when necessary), and rid them of the anxiety of having a chronic incurable disease, allowing them to return to the quality of life they deserve. The teaching of IBS related matters should constitute at least a three-hour curriculum for medical students. In academic centers' GI Departments, IBS needs to be taken more seriously. IBS should no longer be considered a simple patient problem, just a number to be seen by a nurse practitioner (NP) and/or physician assistant (PA). Instead, it should be seen as an issue worthy of a comprehensive consultation by a knowledgeable physician devoted to seeing these patients. Several case histories of patients seen and treated by me, and described at the end of this book will illustrate my point.

In this book, I have tried to help educate you about your problems and their potential causes, in order to prepare you for your doctor visit. Hopefully, this material will allow you to have an intelligent conversation with your health care provider, and help you to know how to ask for a proper diagnostic evaluation in order to find the etiology/reasons behind your problems, finally leading to relief from your long standing IBS symptoms "for good".

Please note that this book is a general guide for patients suffering from IBS symptoms. It doesn't replace seeking the immediate advice of a gastroenterologist. This is especially true if Alarm symptoms are present, or if symptoms start after age 40, or have been there for a short duration. Since IBS is often a lifelong problem and it starts from early age, it can be chronic and intermittent. If symptoms are short in duration, intensify over time, include blood in the stool, or are associated with weight loss, it is likely an organic disease and deserves the immediate attention of a health care professional.

Alarm symptoms include early satiety, poor appetite, weight loss of more than 10% of body weight, anemia, blood in the stool (whether visible or occult), abdominal pain that increases in intensity over time that is present daily, continuing and worsening diarrhea, new onset constipation, being age 50 or older, and a family history of colitis, Crohn's, celiac disease, colon cancer or polyps, etc.

PATHOPHYSIOLOGY OF IBS

It is out of the scope of this book to delve deeply into the patho-physiology of IBS. However, I'll point out some highlights of con-ventional wisdom indicating the evolution of the thought process from mid-20th century onward regarding abnormal gut motility, visceral hypersensitivity, brain-gut interaction and 5HT mediated sensitivity. Gut microbiome dysbiosis and bile acid imbalance play an important part in the pathophysiology of IBS.

Beginning in the 1940s, an enormous body of literature has been published that extensively characterizes traditional factors believed to be involved in the genesis of symptoms, including motor, sensory, central nervous system and psychological abnormalities.

The enteric (ENS) nervous system, like the central nervous sys-tem (CNS), has integrated circuits for feedback, reflexes, and infor-mation processing. Disregulation of CNS-ENS interaction causes visceral hypersensitivity and abnormal colonic motility (hallmarks of functional GI disorders).

Because IBS symptoms are the result of multiple causes, it's likely that these factors participate to varying degrees in different patients. For example, patients with IBS show exaggerated colon motor responsiveness to exogenous stimulation, including abnor-mally prolonged and intense colonic contractions after colorectal balloon inflation, cholinergic stimulation and colon perfusion of deoxycholicacid (bile acid). However, many of the distal gut symp-toms in IBS~C may relate to anorectal outlet dysfunction rather than colon abnormalities.

The serotonin pathway plays an important role in modulating-gut motility. Serotonin (5HT) is a neurotransmitter in both the gut and the brain at every level, and has a role in mediating visceral hyper sensitivity and the peristaltic reflex. 95% of 5HT is found in the gut, with 90% localized within enterochromaffin cells of the intestinal mucosa (lining). It has been reported that IBS patients have higher post-prandial levels of serotonin, and that they remain higher for longer periods of time.

As with motor abnormalities, alterations in visceral and somatic perception are prevalent in IBS patients. Abdominal sensations are mediated by afferent pathways activated by stimuli acting on mechanoreceptors (which detect changes in tension), mesenteric nociceptors (which detect painful stimuli), and chemoreceptors (which senses stool osmolarity, temperature, and pH). Information from these receptors is transmitted by afferent pathways to the brain, where conscious perception occurs. Hypersensitivity may present as hyperalgesia (increase in pain intensity reporting for a given painful stimulus compared with a controlled population), allodynia (reporting of pain from a stimulus not considered painful by healthy individuals), and exaggerated pain referral pattern (perception of pain outside the normal anatomic sites, normally not felt in healthy individuals). In a substantial number of patients with IBS, pain is experienced at lower volumes or pressures from rectal or ileal balloon inflation than healthy controls.

Some patients suffering IBS-C, with hard stools, and no fecal urgency, show reduced perceptual responses to rectal distending balloon stimuli.

Patients with IBS also may show atypical pain referral patterns during gut distension stimuli, reporting pain diffusely in the abdomen, back, shoulder, or chest.

Colonic hypersensitivity is augmented by ingestion of cold water and high-fat meals, especially in IBS-D. Repeated sigmoid colon distentions produce prominent hyperalgesia, as well as abnormal pain referral patterns in IBS. Some investigators attribute exaggerated pain perception in IBS to psychological factors. IBS patients have a stronger tendency to report sensations as painful or a negative experience during gut distention versus controls.

A study of rectal gas inflation reported increases in perception of bloating in IBS patients associated with changes in external and internal oblique muscle contraction, indicating an interaction of visceral and somatic musculature in production of gaseous symptomatology. Individuals with IBS-D show abnormal sympathetic adrenergic activity. Conversely, individuals with IBS-C show vagus parasympathetic dysfunction as measured by heart rate variability profile. A study also showed persistence of autonomic defects, even during sleep in IBS patients, suggesting that they are intrinsic characteristics of the disease rather than consequentes of psychosocial influences.

However, in spite of all above mentioned studies, it is noteworthy that:

- Although motor abnormalities of the GI tract (increased frequency and irregularities of luminal contractions, abnormal transit time) are detected in some patients, no predominant pattern has emerged as a marker for IBS.

- Selective hyper sensitization of visceral afferent nerves in the gut has been observed.

- In some patients with IBS, mucosal immune system activation is seen (post infectious gastroenteritis IBS).

- Changes in fecal microflora are getting more attention.

- Food specific antibodies in some patients may have a role.

- Diet-induced carbohydrate malabsorption, in my opinion, is the major contributor to bloating, gas and irregular BM.

- Gluten sensitivity and gut permeability (leaky gut) are getting more attention.

- Genetic susceptibility may be a factor.

- Psychological factors: patients with IBS have more anxiety, depression, phobia, somatization and sleep problems.

- Bile acid-induced IBS-D, either primary or secondary, warrant more examination when evaluating IBS patients.

A study of fecal biomarkers showed that in 73% of IBS-D patients there is low growth of beneficial bacteria (Lactobacillus & Bifidobacterium) and increased Veillonella spp in IBS-C groups.

Bile acid levels were increased in the stool of 25% of IBS-D patients, and decreased in IBS-C patients.

Increased amounts of the eosinophils protein x in 14% of patients suggested food allergies or parasites, while high levels of the white blood cell protein calprotectin in 12% of patients indicated inflammation, and decreased levels of pancreatic elastase in 7% was due to pancreatic insufficiency. Parasites were found in 7% of patients.

IBS SYMPTOMS

S ince there is no diagnostic test for IBS, the Rome Foundation started categorizing functional GI disorders, IBS included.

For diagnosing IBS, **Rome II** criteria was defined as "at least 12 weeks, which need not be consecutive, in the preceding 12 months of abdominal discomfort that has two out of three features: 1) related to defecation, 2) onset associated with a change in frequency or form and 3) appearance of stool"

Supportive symptoms include an abnormal stool frequency of more than three bowel movements a day or less than three bowel movements a week, stool form which is lumpy, hard or watery, passage associated with straining, urgency, or a feeling of incomplete evacuation, passage of mucus, bloating or a feeling of abdominal distention.

The most recent **Rome IV** criteria for IBS is simplified as recurrent abdominal pain, on average, at least one day per week in the last three months, associated with two or more of the following criteria related to defecation, associated with change in stool frequency, or change in stool form (appearance).

Manning criteria for IBS include: pain relief with defecation, more frequent stool at the onset of pain, looser stool at the onset of pain, visible abdominal distention, passage of mucus, sensation of incomplete evacuation. The likelihood of IBS is proportional to the number of Manning criteria that are present.

1/4 of IBS patients are constipated, 1/4 have diarrhea, and half of them have a combination of diarrhea and constipation (more in females).

IBS is characterized by chronic abdominal discomfort, gas, bloating and altered bowel habits. Pain is of a visceral type, and may be due to stretching and tension on the intestinal walls and the effect of noxious stimuli affecting mechanical and chemoreceptors. Pain may be crampy, with variable intensity and periodic exacerbation. Emotional stress and diet may exacerbate the pain. Patients often complain about excess bloating, flatulence and burping. Normal bowel movements with periods of diarrhea and constipation are also common. Bloating, gas and irregular bowel habits are the most common complaints of IBS patients that I see in my office.

IBS diarrhea (IBS-D) typically entails frequent loose bowel movements, in small amounts, during waking hours (mostly in the morning), preceded by urgency and abdominal distress. IBS diarrhea is osmotic, with a pH less than six, and less than 50% increased mucus. However, in one study of non-constipated females with IBS, 36% had abdominal discomfort, 28% experienced urgency, 12% had bloating, 22% reported a change of bowel movements, and only 1% had mucus in the stool.

IBS patients often have both hard and loose stools over periods of hours, days, weeks or months. Subtypes may vary, suggesting changes in diet.

IBS should only be diagnosed in the absence of structural or metabolic abnormalities. Additionally, both normal and abnormal food-related reactions can cause some or all of IBS-like symptoms. Please keep in mind that in a significant number of patients, more than one reason could be contributing collectively to induce different symptoms with different intensity from day to day depending on circumstances. In this case, correcting one or two issues may not be enough to eliminate symptoms completely.

BRISTOL STOOL CHART

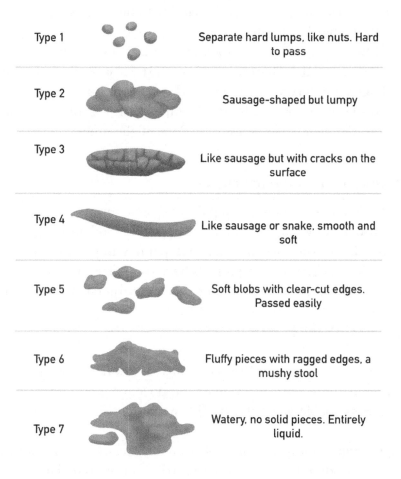

Type 1	Separate hard lumps, like nuts. Hard to pass
Type 2	Sausage-shaped but lumpy
Type 3	Like sausage but with cracks on the surface
Type 4	Like sausage or snake, smooth and soft
Type 5	Soft blobs with clear-cut edges. Passed easily
Type 6	Fluffy pieces with ragged edges, a mushy stool
Type 7	Watery, no solid pieces. Entirely liquid.

Bristol stool form correlates with intestinal transit time and contents.

Type 1 - separate hard lumps

Type 2 - sausage shape but lumpy

Type 3 - sausage shape but cracks on edges

Type 4 - like sausage or snake smooth and soft
Type 5 - soft blobs with clear cut edges
Type 6 - mushy stool
Type 7 - watery with non-solid pieces

The latest classification of IBS includes 4 phenotypes.

IBS-C: hard or lumpy stools at least 25% of the time

IBS-D: loose or watery stools at least 25% of the times

IBS-M: hard or lumpy stools at least 25% of the times and loose or watery stools at least 25% of the times

IBS-U (unsubtyped): hard or lumpy stools less than 25% and loose or watery stools less than 25% of the times

DIARRHEA CLASSIFICATIONS

Fatty diarrhea: stool is bulky, pale, and malodorous

Inflammatory diarrhea: liquid stools with blood and mucus

Osmotic diarrhea: less than 200 ML per day, improves or resolves with fasting, most IBS patients have osmotic diarrhea

Secretory diarrhea: large volume, watery, and persist during fasting

ALARM SYMPTOMS

Patients presenting with IBS symptoms, if they have any of the following features, must be evaluated at once for other more serious maladies capable of producing IBS symptoms.

- Signs and symptoms of iron deficiency anemia and/or blood in the stools, either visible or occult (Guaiac, FIT)

- Unintentional weight loss, 10% or more of body weight

- Palpable abdominal mass or enlarge lymph nodes on physical exam

- Family history of colon cancer that has not had age-appropriate colonoscopy screening

- Onset of symptoms more than age 50, with no prior screening colonoscopy

- Sudden or acute onset of new change in bowel habits

- Short duration with worsening symptoms

- Family history of Crohn's, ulcerative colitis, or Celiac Sprue

HRQL IN IBS
(Health-related quality of life)

HRQL is measured or defined by the extent to which one's usual or expected physical, emotional and social well-being are affected by a medical condition or its treatment (this criteria is subjective and multidimensional). Because of subjectivity, individuals have different expectations and coping abilities while having the same medical issue. Therefore, HRQL must be measured from individual viewpoint rather than that of outside observers. The importance of obtaining HRQL reports from patient is due to disparate estimates of symptoms and HRQL between what patients feel and what their physician perceives.

Multi-dimensionality framework HRQL is divided into physical, mental, and social health. Subcomponents of mental health are comprised of anxiety, depression, cognitive function, experience of stress, psychological impact, or even resultant smoking, drinking and addiction.

IBS patients have the same HRQL as patients with diabetes mellitus and lower than patients with GERD and depression. Also, mental HRQL scores are lower than in patients with chronic renal failure. The health utility of severe IBS is similar to class 3 congestive heart failure. When evaluating and measuring HRQL in IBS patients, one must ask about feeling and degree of pain, general health perception, energy level, social functioning, emotional well-being, sexual function, health worries, body image, bowel symptoms, and sleep disturbances due to IBS.

A BRIEF DESCRIPTION OF GI TRACT ANATOMY, PHYSIOLOGY, FUNCTION AND PATHOPHYSIOLOGY AS IT RELATES TO CAUSING IBS-SIMILAR SYMPTOMS

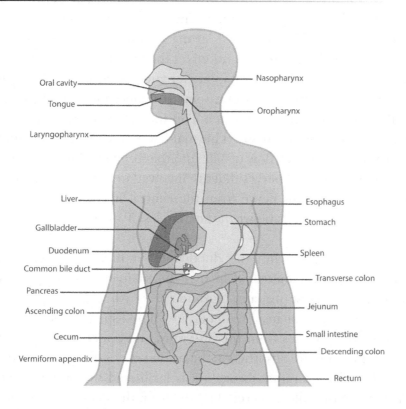

The GI tract is a tube that starts from the mouth and end in the anus. In addition, The liver, gall bladder and pancreas are part of the GI system.

In the oral cavity, the food is chewed. It is then mixed with sal-ivary juice that contains amylase, which breaks down starch, and lingual lipase, which break downs fat.

Then the food bolus is swallowed, and the esophagus propels food down into the stomach. There is a valve between the esopha-gus and the stomach that stays closed all of the time, except when we start swallowing, This valve opens to allow food and liquids into the stomach, and releases air and depressurizes when full. If this valve malfunctions, we will suffer from gastroesophageal reflux and its consequences. The stomach's main enzyme is pep-sin, which breaks down proteins. Meanwhile, gastric acid breaks down food fibers and eliminates any bacteria entering the stom-ach. The stomach also has a strong peristaltic contraction that mechanically breaks down and mixes the food and, when ready, it pushes it through the pyloric sphincter and pyloric channel into the duodenum. During endoscopy, some patients show patent pylorus with a malfunctioning sphincter. This may allow food to enter the duodenum before it's ready. This maldigestion can cause bloating, and also allow a back flow of bile into the stomach. There are mul-tiple hormones and nerves that are involved in peristaltic function, including the vagus nerve from the central nervous system, and myenteric nerve cells between the muscles of the GI tract.

While food reaches the duodenum, it mixes with enzymes secreted by the pancreas, which is the main source of enzymes necessary to digest proteins, fats and carbohydrates. The pancreas is also the source of insulin that adjusts blood sugar. Protein needs endo/exopeptidases from the intestines and pancreas in order to digest. Proteins are absorbed in the brush border of the small intes-tine. Fat digestion and absorption is facilitated by the pancreatic enzyme lipase. Bile is secreted by the liver, then concentrated and stored in the gallbladder. It then enters the duodenum along with fatty foods. Therefore, fat absorption requires the pancreas (lipoly-sis), liver (bile salts), intestinal cells (absorption) and lymphatic cells (transport). Carbohydrates (starch, sugar, lactose) require pancre-atic amylase to convert to maltose. Maltose, sucrose and lactose are absorbed in the brush border of the small bowel by their respective enzymes maltase, sucrase, and lactase. However, fructose, the main sugar in fruits (even though it is a monosaccharide) can't enter intestinal cells independently, and needs to piggy-back on glucose. Intestinal epithelial cells are renewed and turned over every 48–72 hours. In fact, the bowel ages very well, there is very little change in its capacity for digestion and absorption as we get older. After the food is ready to be absorbed, the intestinal cells and their villi will absorb the food in the form of glucose, fructose and galactose for carbohydrates. They are carried via the portal vein into the liver and into general circulation. The liver stores extra sugar as glycogen to be released when necessary. If the liver's capacity is too low for this storage, the sugar turns glucose and fructose into undesirable fat. Triglycerides in genetically susceptible persons can cause fatty liver, NASH hepatitis and even cirrhosis and liver cancer. However, fat globules use the lymphatic system to bypass the liver to reach all of the cells throughout the body, so the source of fatty liver is not dietary fat or cholesterol. The small intestine can only absorb carbs in the form of monosaccharides, and also has an active part in digesting lactose. Lactase stored in brush borders breaks down milk sugar lactose into galactose and glucose. Brush border enzyme maltase converts maltose into 2 glucose, and sucrase breaks down the table sugar into glucose and fructose. Glucose absorption has an active mechanism, but fructose piggy-backs itself on glucose to get absorbed. After all digested foods, fluids and electrolytes are absorbed some fluids and residual stuff that was not digestible in the small intestine enters the colon.

The large intestine stores waste, but, more importantly, it absorbs water and electrolytes that remain in the contents that enter it, and has a very active and important **MICROBIOME** residing in it that functions to take up the food that was unable to be digested in the small intestine. Then bacteria works on the part of the food that is fermentable and digestible. The bacteria digests these parts and produces calories, as well as useful fatty acids taken up by large intestinal cells as a nutrient. This process produces gases (mostly carbon dioxide, hydrogen, and methane). Of course, the gas that exits the anus also contains some nitrogen and oxygen, which is the residual of what was swallowed in the form of air. Usually 25 to 30% of flatus is swallowed air.

Depending on the type of diet, diarrhea in IBS may last for a few hours, days or weeks. It may be temporarily replaced by constipation, and then return. It may be associated with mid to lower abdominal cramps, bloating, and excessive gas. As an example of chronic persistent cases, consider celiac disease in the Western hemisphere. Celiac sprue may just present as iron deficiency anemia. Even those with known celiac that are following a gluten-free diet should be aware that many foods (including frozen custard, instant coffee and even ketchup) have added gluten. Some over-the-counter medications (including dietary supplements, magnesium tablets, certain antacids and even sorbitol in sugar-free chewing gum) can cause cramps and mucus diarrhea that passes quickly, as can improperly absorbed food, excessive bile acid loss to the colon, food allergies, thyroid disease, and laxative abuse. In some patients suffering from anxiety, distress and mood disturbances can create similar symptoms. Stressful situations like exam times, meeting the parents of your significant other, interviewing for a new job, remembering childhood stressful events, conflicts with a spouse at home, repeated sexual or emotional abuse, being bullied in the school, being pushed too hard to excel or long forgotten stressors related to past experiences can also influence our GI tract. Discussing them with a professional psychotherapist for a few sessions may help. When experiencing diarrhea associated with spasm and discomfort in the left lower quadrant, these symptoms may improve with fiber supplements, which not only absorb excess mucus but also fill the sigmoid colon, preventing any excess squeeze on it (the empty tooth paste tube analogy).

INTESTINAL MICROBIOME

Intestinal microbiome is an important auxiliary and virtual organ, it plays an important role in energy harvest, storage and expenditure.

The human body has 10 times more bacteria than cells. Without these bacteria, we would be undernourished. Microbiome bacteria breaks down undigested carbohydrate and fat. Indeed, the large intestine is a bioreactor in which the host uses bacteria to degrade indigestible leftovers. Bacteria produce calories and valuable substances such as vitamin K and vitamin B. They also metabolize drugs and toxins, and produce short chain fatty acids (SCFAs), which are the necessary nutrients for colon epithelial cells, and also function as a barrier for pathogenic bacteria. Bacteria are also responsible for reduction in fecal mass. Most bacteria in the colon are anaerobes. There are 3000 to 5000 bacterial species in the colon. 90% of fecal mass is bacteria, and concentrations are up to 10 billion bacteria per gram of stool. They actively multiply. What facilitates their growth is peristaltic movements which massage stool, thereby mixing bacteria with nutrients, fibers and undigested food. This process helps to maintain optimal viscosity and temperature for these bacteria.

More than 50 phyla have been described; however, only 4 major phyla predominate: Firmicutes, Bacteroidetes, Actinobacteria, and

Proteobacteria. The GI tract is also colonized by fungi and viruses which constitute the gut mycobiome and virome respectively.

Every individual's microbiome is unique, like his/her fingerprint.

70% of bacteria in the colon are habitual bacterias that are present in every person and have been around since the beginning of life. The rest are commensal and mutual bacteria, and include certain bacteria groups like bifidobacteriaceae, enterobacteriaceae, clostridia, lactobacilli, and enterococci, which are often present but not obligatory for the healthy human intestine.

Commensalism is an association between two organisms in which one benefits and the others derives neither benefit nor harm. When they both benefit it is called mutualism.

Commensal and mutual bacteria salvage undigested food in order to produce metabolic energy (2.5–3.1 Kcal per gram), as well as gases (including hydrogen, carbon dioxide and methane) which are all odorless, and short chain fatty acids (butyrate, propionate and acetate).

Considerable amounts of produced organic acid and gases are absorbed by colonic mucosa and the rest are passed as flatus. The major fatty acid produced is butyrate, a main source of nutrition in the gut's epithelium. Butyrate also has anti-inflammatory and immuno-modulatory properties thought to strengthen innate immunity.

Bacteria produce multiple vitamins, antioxidants, beneficial chemicals and toxins to eliminate harmful bacteria. They stimulate production of glutathione, which controls intestinal inflammation, prevents cancer cells from developing, contributes to obesity, and encourages production of hormones for a healthy metabolism. For example, humans provides food and a place to live for E. Coli in the large intestine and in return E. coli produces vitamin K and prevents harmful bacteria from establishing themselves in our colon.

All of the bacteria in our large intestine make it harder for invasive disease-causing pathogens to establish a foothold inside us and cause disease.

Some of the indigenous bacteria in the colon are known pathogens outside of the colon. To name a few: E. coli causes sepsis and urinary tract infection, bacteroids cause abscess, enterococci cause endocarditis and clostridium histolyuticaum causes gas gangrene.

A host tolerates bacteria by separating them from the colon lining with a protective mucus layer. The colon and terminal ileum biopsy from healthy persons are covered with mucus that's free of bacteria; therefore, bacteria are never found in direct contact with intestinal cells and crypts.

The mucus has 3 layers like onion skin, and each layer has different viscosity due to degrees of dehydration. Mucus is continuously renewed and the part attached to intestinal lining cells has the most viscosity, and bacteria can't penetrate it. Next to it is a mucus layer that is less viscous (the germinal zone of mucus) that holds the blue print of an individual's microbiome (biofilm mass). This layer regenerates microbiome mass after clearing the colon when preparing for colonoscopy or after acute gastroenteritis. The 3rd mucus layer is least viscous. It covers and lubricates stool for ease of passage.

If the mucus layer is disturbed and bacteria contact and enter enterocytes, it causes inflammation, crypt abscess, ulcers or fissures. 90% of the bacteria found in the mucus of patients with inflammation are habitual bacteria. Bacteria in the biofilm mass in inflammatory bowel disease are more than 50% bacteriod fragilis. More than 50% of the biofilm mass in irritable bowel syndrome is eubacterium rectale (a major contributor to the production of butyrate), and faccalibacterium prausnitzii, an anti-inflammatory bacterium. Whereas, in patients with inflammatory bowel disease, these bacteria are less than 30%. Studies show that there is even a relationship between gut microbiome and responses to different treatment in IBD. The more beneficial bacteria, the better response. The more E.Coli, the less favorable response.

Lack of exposure to different bacteria due to high hygiene, exposure to bacteria imported from a different region of the world, substances that reduce viscosity of the mucus barrier like detergents and emulsifiers, bile salts, gluten, cigarette smoking, and defensin (host defense peptides) can all reduce the viscosity of mucus barriers and allow for a disease state to develop.

Diarrhea of any cause is associated with increased thickness of the mucus layer and growing mucus in the fecal mass, except in ulcerative colitis patients, in which case the mucus layer is depleted.

In diarrhea, the habitual bacteria in the center of feces is reduced or destroyed, but bacteria in the germinal zone biofilm of mucus remains the same, and proportional to previously healthy stool. That's why with colonoscopy prep or diarrheal disease colon bacteria returns to it's normal state in a short period of time. In patients with active Crohn's disease, there is a complete depletion of F. prausnitzii from the central and germinal zones of feces.

The gut microbiota of individuals is dominated by different fiber utilizing bacteria which ferment dietary fiber into short chain fatty acids known to be important in human health.

Human gut microbiome, although unique to each person like his/her fingerprints, all fall into one of three major groups called Enterotypes, based on bacteria predominance for fiber fermentation. Enterotype 1 is associated with a Western diet, which is dominated by bacteroides that produce more propionate.

Enterotype 2 is prevotella dominant (bacteroidia).

EnteroType 3, or the grain lovers enterotype, is dominated by ruminococcus and bifidobacterium. Long-term eating habits of this group include consuming resistant starches and dietary fiber.

Obesity is associated with a high number of firmicutes and lower number of bacterioidetes. They extract more calories from fermentable foods (undigestable part of fruits and vegetables). Indeed, High-FODMAP foods are a prebiotic source of energy for these bacteria. Enterotype 2 correlates with low level of microbiota previously associated with immune regulating properties. More than 40 different prevotella species exist with highly different behavior. Enterotype 3 produces more butyrate than other SCFAs. Butyrate has beneficial anti-inflammatory and immunomodulary effects.

Some foods like apples, barley, garlic, oats, onion, and flax seed will help increase firmicutes bacteria resulting more in beneficial butyrate.

A Western diet that is high in fat, animal proteins and sugar has negative effects on these beneficial grain lovers gut bacteria.

Methanogens are archaea that produce methane under anaerobic conditions. Methane is in the belches of ruminants and in the flatulence of humans.

Methane-producing archaea are abundant in obese humans and mice. Methanogen bacteria oxidize hydrogen produced by fermentation of undigested carbohydrates, to produce methane (CH_4), leading to higher production and absorption of short chain fatty acid which may lead to obesity. Also they reduces bloating and flatulence by reducing hydrogen volume (4 Hydrogen atoms in a molecule of methane). Methane is eliminated by 80% through flatus, and 20% is excreted by the lungs. Methane causes constipation by slowing intestinal transit time.

Long term changes in diet affect enterotype, but temporary changes in diet only temporarily affect composition within 24 hours to facilitate fermentation benefits.

Intestinal Microbiome changes with age. As an infant grows into adulthood, the dominance of firmicutes and bifidobacterium is replaced by bacteroides and prevotella. Healthy adults have more lactobacillus acidophilus and helveticus, and elderly people have more lactobacillus plantarum, lactobacillus paracasei and L. reteri. Diversity of bacterial species is reduced in elderly. There is a decline in the beneficial function of gut microbiota, and an increase in inflammatory and disease producing bacteria, especially in individuals over 90 years old. In the elderly, two major microbial phyla firmicutes and bacteroides represent 99% of bacteria in their guts. There is a significant decrease in useful bifidobacterium and lactobacilli with aging.

There is also an age-related increase in facultative anaerobes (which can become aerobe and use oxygen as well) such as streptococci, enterococci, and enterobacteria, which are capable of becoming pathogens when outside the gut.

There is a paucity of lactobacilli and bifidobacteria species in the stool of IBS patients. I suspect one reason may be that more than 60% of IBS patients have lactose intolerance and avoid eating dairy foods, especially milk, which is prebiotic for these beneficial bacteria.

IBS constipation patients have increased methane-producing ruminococcus. Protebacteria or pseudomonata are associated with metabolic syndrome and inflammation, obesity, diabetes, fatty liver and NASH. Some are pathogens if they enter the GI tract, like some Escherichia, Salmonella, Vibrio and Yersinia.

Some studies have indicated the following interesting points: Ruminococcus, Eubacterium and Fecalibacterium produce butyr ate, which has anti-inflammatory effects. A fiber-enriched diet with fruits and vegetables reduces risk of inflammatory bowel disease. A vegetarian diet and lacto-ovo-vegetarian diet with fish once a week and red meat every two weeks prevent relapses of Crohn's disease. High fiber diets reduce asthma attacks and recurring bronchitis in children. A high-fat diet reduces bacterioedates and increases firmicutes bacteria. Animal fat increase bacteroides.

MALDIGESTION AND MALABSORPTION

There are a number of significant gastrointestinal problems that can produce symptoms that mimic IBS, and they need to be ruled out before a diagnosis of IBS is made.

In over half a century of being an MD with extensive clinical experience, I have rarely seen patients that I was convinced truly had IBS. Almost all of my patients who were diagnosed with IBS, or complained of multiple symptoms, have had one or several issues related to digestion and absorption, and improved with different dietary changes and/or appropriate medical treatment of the causes of their symptoms.

To familiarize readers, first I will begin with a very brief explanation of normal digestion and absorption, and the conditions that may produce one or several symptoms of IBS, starting from the beginning of the GI tract (the mouth) to the end (the anus).

In the oral cavity, chewing properly and thoroughly and eating slowly is important. The digestion and absorption of simple carbohydrates starts in the mouth chewing, mixing and salivary glands amylase. Eating in a hurry and swallowing too much air, or reduced saliva causing dry mouth can contribute to bloating.

The esophagus carries the food bolus down into the stomach. Some patients may have poor peristalsis and/or incompetent LES, and suffer from gastroesophageal reflux.

In the stomach, food is broken down by strong gastric mixing contractions, propulsing peristalsis, gastric acid, and proteolytic enzymes. Poor peristalsis, hypo acidity—either due to medications like too much Omeprazole or intrinsic like atrophic gastritis—will present with early satiety, postprandial bloating, nausea and anorexia. This is seen mostly in patients with diabetes, patients taking strong doses of PPIs to control reflux, or chronic gastritis due to helicobacter pylori.

Once food enters the duodenum, it is digested mainly by the pancreatic enzymes amylase, lipase and proteases, and small intestinal brush border enzymes that break down lactose and table sugar.

Fat digestion and absorption is facilitated by lipase secreted into the small intestine by the pancreas and bile from the liver. Any problems in the pancreas (like chronic pancreatitis caused by too much alcohol drinking), recurrent acute pancreatitis, etc., or intestinal brush border enzymes deficiency (such as lactase deficiency or sucrase-iso maltase deficiency will cause improper digestion and residual undi gested food gets carried to the colon.

Small intestinal bacterial overgrowth (SIBO) is caused by a number of different problems, including poor peristalsis, small bowel diverticulosis, adhesions causing localized narrowing of small intestine and Crohn's disease. SIBO can cause overgrowth of bacteria in the small intestine and interfere with normal digestion and absorption and cause bloating, diarrhea, and abdominal discomfort. The environment in the small intestine becomes like that of the colon, with too many bacteria present that ferment normal food that has not yet been absorbed.

Leaky gut syndrome (in the small intestine), due to multiple reasons such as medications or food allergies, can cause IBS symptoms.

Once the food reaches large intestine, undigested and unabsorbed but fermentable food residue (FODMAP) will be consumed by the large intestinal bacteria capable of breaking them down and consuming them as nutrients. The undigested food presented to the colon, depending on quantity, may cause loose stool (osmotic diarrhea), and the gases produce bloating and abdominal distention. Therefore, depending on many factors, such as the type of diet, amount of undigested food that gets presented to the large intestine, the kind and amount of bacteria that are present in the large intestine, the speed of fermentation, intestinal peristalsis, the capacity of the large intestine to handle the gas, psychological issues, whether the patient able to have a bowel movement when "Mother Nature" calls, or even whether the patient feels free at work or home to get rid of retained gas as flatus can all be responsible for a variety of presentations with different symptoms and intensity (diarrhea, bloating, pain) depending on the day.

Constipated patients may have more symptoms because osmotic materials that produce gas are being retained in the back of an already full colon with poor function. Depending on the substrate, a constipated patient may have a normal bowel movement one day and diarrhea the next if too much FODMAP has entered the colon.

Constipation itself could be due to slow transit and poor peristalsis in the colon, a dilated colon with weak muscle or intrinsic nervous system problems, non-functional or dyssynergic pelvic floor abnormalities causing difficulty coordinating anal sphincter relaxation when nature calls to have a bowel movement, or weak abdominal wall and pelvic floor muscles. Also, not being in the proper psychosocial space or having proper time can delay having a bowel movement, which leads to drying stool in the rectum, thereby increasing symptoms accordingly.

Type and amount of food consumption (namely carbohydrates, fat, fruits and vegetables), too much fructose, gluten in those with gluten sensitivity or gluten allergy, lactose in dairy products if lactase deficiency is present, food allergies of different kinds (but mostly IgG related) can cause bloating, diarrhea, and abdominal discomfort. Many different medications can interfere with proper digestion, absorption, peristalsis or microbiome and can produce symptoms similar to IBS.

Multiple gastrointestinal surgical procedures can be solely responsible for symptoms of diarrhea, bloating, abdominal discomfort, etc.

From this brief description, one can realize that there are many conditions causing "IBS" symptoms and they need to be ruled out carefully before patients are committed to a wrong diagnosis with lifelong symptoms, QoL issues and unnecessary medication use.

GAS & BLOATING

Large Capacity to Expand	Small Capacity to Expand
Male	Female

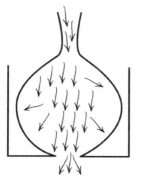 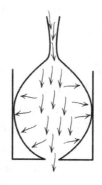

Large Amounts of Gas Expands Intestine No Symptoms	Even Small Amounts of Gas Causes Feelings of Bloating & Discomfort

Feeling puffed up, having a noisy stomach, bowel gas/flatus and belching are by far the most common GI complaints. Frequent belching, even though annoying, is due to swallowing too much air and not necessarily a sign of disease. However, stomach distention and bloating, acid reflux, PPI use, aerophagia, chronic gastritis, or drinking carbonated beverages and beer can cause belching (swallowing too much air).In some cultures, a necessary and obligatory post prandial belch is a sign of enjoying the meal and thanking the host or God for a delicious meal.

Bloat s the sensation of having a bowel full of gas and blowing up. Patients experiencing bloating complain of clothes feeling tight and/or passing flatus frequently. They may have lower abdominal discomfort, diarrhea and constipation or both. Evidence suggests that gut motor and sensory dysfunction, as well as somatic factors. participate in the sensation of bloating. IBS-C patients are more bloated because of delay in colon and small intestine transit time. Patients with IBS report a greater degree of symptoms with a similar amount of gas retention. With similar total intestinal gas volume, people report different degrees of symptoms.

Keep in mind that in females feeling bloated, it may be related to problems with ovaries (cancer), and the uterus (menstrual period or endometriosis). In chronic alcoholics, cirrhosis of the liver can cause fluid retention and ascites, creating a distended abdomen and the feeling of being bloated.

Excessive flatus: excess gastrointestinal gas occurs for several reasons, including excessive air swallowing, fast eating, carbonated beverages, beer drinking, excessive FODMAP foods, SIBO, carbohydrate maldigestion and malabsorption due to inborn errors of metabolism like lactase deficiency, diseases of the pancreas and small bowel causing maldigestion and malabsorption, multiple known medications, etc. These factors can result in the production of large amounts of hydrogen, carbon dioxide, and methane gases in addition to swallowed air. Foul smelling gas is often due to undigested proteins containing sulfur, broccoli, cabbage, beans, onion, garlic, too much fat and fried foods. Most normal people pass flatus at least 20 times daily. If experiencing recent excesses, or if associated with diarrhea and abdominal pain, see a physician to look for the cause. There could be several. Treatment of too much gas, bloating and flatus is incremental and begins with restricting FODMAP, lactose and carbohydrates in the patient's diet, prescribing antibiotics if SIBO is suspected, implementing the trial of a gluten-free diet, a pancreatic enzyme supplement for improving digestion of fat and carbohydrates, taking Gas-X, Lactaid milk and Lactaid pills with dairy, using Beano with beans and legumes, or taking activated charcoal with chlorophyl tablets. The patient can treat beans by boiling them for 3 minutes and leaving them in the same water overnight, then washing them the next day. This will eliminate most of the gas source of beans. If constipation occurs, manage it with appropriate medications. Probiotics are recommended, but, in my experience, they are not worth the price.

Volatile sulfur containing substrates from proteins is malodorous due to bacterial metabolite of proteins.

Hydrogen sulfide smells like rotten egg, and Fraternity hall smells like rotten cabbage and garlic. One study found that men fart 2–53 times a day with an average of 12.7 times. Women 1 to 32 times a day with average of 7.1 times. The number of farts was higher when people ate more fiber. Also farts contain volatile sulfur com pounds and molecules like indole and skatole, which are often linked to the smell of feces. In people eating pinto beans or baked beans daily, half of them fart more and when they continue to eat beans after a few weeks farting becomes less frequently and nears normal.

Holding on to gas for too long can cause abdominal pain, and IBS-like symptoms in susceptible individuals. Contrary to popular belief, taking activated charcoal pills four times daily doesn't change the volume or smell of farts. Avoiding dietary fibers reduces gas, but soluble fibers, like oat, decrease colorectal cancer, hemorrhoids and diverticulosis. So, if gas doesn't cause pain for you, most of the times it is healthy, and those around you may just have to learn to "turn the other cheek."

The age old wise tale for children to eat their beans

Beans, beans, the musical fruit
The more you eat, the more you toot
The more you toot, the better you feel
So lift your leg and let them squeal!

Another version

Beans, beans, they are good for your heart
The more you eat, the more you fart
The more you fart, the better you feel
So eat those beans at every meal!

In conclusion, in a healthy person with no evidence of GI tract disease, having gas is normal and healthy and it indicates eating food high in prebiotics.

If and when you feel uncomfortable, like when meeting a date or other social events, you may achieve comfort by avoiding high-FODMAP foods, lactose and gluten to achieve a desirable comfort and acceptable level of gas.

PSEUDO-IBS

In this section I will describe a variety of conditions that can cause symptoms similar to IBS. Patients are often diagnosed with IBS without really having IBS. I call it Pseudo-IBS, and this is the main reason for writing this book. It is the physician's duty, and the patient's responsibility to make sure that the following conditions have been ruled out before a diagnosis of IBS is made.

IBS is described as specific symptoms of change in bowel habits (shape and number), and abdominal discomfort that changes with bowel movement, one or two days a week for 3 months of the last 12 months. This description begs the question of symptoms being related to some, most likely, dietary exposures that may happen on and off, and patients are often not aware of nor informed of their diet being the cause of their IBS-like symptoms.

DIFFERENTIAL DIAGNOSIS OF CAUSES OF IBS-LIKE SYMPTOMS

The followings can cause all or some symptoms that puts patients in the category of IBS; therefore, it's important to rule them out prior to accepting IBS as your diagnosis and thereby leaving you with its consequences of long-term discomfort, medications and interference with your quality of life (QoL)

High-FODMAP diet

Carbohydrate intolerance

Lactose intolerance (25% US, 75% world, 60% IBS patients)

Fructose malabsorption and intolerance (30% of people tolerate a limit 25 g per day)

Food intolerance (allergy, non-allergy, alcohol, caffeine, MSG)

Celiac sprue (4.6% IBS patients in US)

SIBO (4% IBS in US)

Achlorhydria, Hypochlorhydria either primary or secondary to chronic PPI use in patients suffering from severe acid reflux

Bile Acids diarrhea that may be due to primary overproduction or Ileal malabsorption, and/or secondary due to malabsorption (SIBO, post Gall bladder removal, ileal resection and short bowel)

Post-surgical (Nissen's fundoplication, gastric sleeve and gastric bypass surgery, small intestinal resection, removal of the cecum and Terminal ileum for cecal and proximal right colon cancer, removal of terminal ileum for Crohn's stricture, fistulae or abscess, intra-abdominal adhesions causing intestinal stricture and partial blockage with stasis, intra-abdominal infections adjacent to a small bowel loops like chronic diverticulitis, etc.)

Chronic Pancreatitis (alcohol, recurrent acute pancreatitis)

GI infection (blastocystis hominis, giardiasis, amoebiasis)

Post gastroenteritis (C-difficile, Campylobacter, Aeromonas, Plesiomonas, etc.)

Medication desired effects and side effects (Olmesartan, Metformin, Acarbose, SSRI, NSAIDs, Antacids, Trulicity, Narcotics, PPIs, etc.)

Enteric neuropathy and myopathy (diabetes mellitus, gastroparesis, SIBO, etc.)

Rapid intestinal transit time

Chronic pancreatitis (alcoholics)

Idiopathic constipation

Hyper or Hypo-Thyroidism

Inflammatory bowel disease (IBD)

Microscopic colitis (5% of IBS-D)

GI malignancies esspically pancreas and colon

Alcohol intolerance

Salicylates sensitivity (all dried fruits, berries, grape, date, cherries, pepper, tomatoes apricots are high in salicylates). Salicylates sensitive patients 78% have IBS-like symptoms, 20% asthma, 60% itching, rash, headache or migraine

Functional GI disorders

Leaky Gut Syndrome (Ehler Donlos syndrome, HIV, Autoimmune Enteritis, Crohn's, Marathon runners, Chronic NSAID use, etc.)

Mast Cell Hyperactivity Syndrome

Candida Albicans overgrowth in stool

Ovarian cancer (bloating and abdominal distention)

Cirrhosis of the liver with ascites (chronic alcoholics with new-onset bloating and abdominal distention)

Other GI disorders like GERD, dyspepsia, Helicobacter pylori-induced gastropathy, biliary dyskinesia and SOD may present with complaints similar to IBS

Multifactorial

The majority of patients with IBS have more than one reason for IBS-like symptoms, and depending on contribution and severity of each problem, a single cause elimination or treatment will result in partial improvement; for example, a patient with celiac sprue also may suffer from lactose intolerance, chronic pancreatitis, auto-immune thyroiditis and SIBO, or an alcoholic drinking a few cans of beer daily may be suffering from gluten sensitivity or celiac, chronic pancreatitis and leaky gut in addition to other causes like lactose intolerance, etc. Or a patient on high-FODMAP food may be suffering from one or more reasons that are causing IBS-similar symptoms. In these instances, eliminating offending foods will only improve IBS symptoms partially.

> My clinical experience is that Carbohydrate-related issues are easily the cause of more than half of pseudo-IBS symptoms, with reasons including a High-FODMAP diet, selective carbohydrate overload, gluten sensitivity, lactose intolerance, fructose overload, etc.

Carbohydrate intolerance mechanism:

Carbohydrates are the mostly available, least expensive, comforting source of humanity's daily caloric intake, and depending on geographic location and culture, it may be mainly bread, pasta, rice, potatoes, fruits, etc.

Carbohydrate issues related to IBS may be from maldigestion to malabsorption related to carbohydrates digestion:

> Inborn or acquired defects of luminal digestion (pancreatic enzymes deficiency) or deficiency of membrane bound intestinal enzymes necessary for digestion of poly-oligo-di-saccharides like lactase deficiency

> Absorption: decreasing absorption of monosaccharides due to a primary defect in mucosal absorption mechanism

(fructose) or secondary to surface reduction from disease or resection

Ingestion of carbohydrates with limited or totally absent digestive and/or absorptive capacity like fructose, mannitol, sorbitol, and dietary fibers

Treatment with lactulose (synthetic dissacharide) and drugs that interfere with carbohydrate absorption like Acarbose, Metformin, and sugar exchange products like sorbitol and fructose

Antibiotics interfering with colonic salvage of malabsorbed or physiologically incompletely absorbed carbohydrates

Food intolerance could be:

- **Quantitative** like taking excessive amount of fructose, fat, gluten, sodas, fibers, and high-FODMAP foods, or

- **Qualitative** like lactose intolerance secondary to lactase deficiency, sucrase-isomaltose deficiency, celiac sprue, food allergy (non-IGA and non-IgE), chronic pancreatitis, status post gastrectomy, cholecystectomy, ileal resection, small bowl narrowing due to adhesions, sleeve gastrectomy, and other conditions that cause SIBO

- Slow transit like diabetic visceral neuropathy, rapid small ball transit time, chronic intestinal Pseudo-obstruction

- Medication like Metformin, Acarbose, NSAID causing both leaky gut and microscopic colitis, chronic PPI use (hypoacidity, bacterial overgrowth and microscopic colitis)

- Poor absorption and rapid transit in Mast cell activation syndrome it present with urticaria, nausea, vomiting, sweating and flushing due to tryptophan and histamine release

- Sucrase-isomaltase deficiency causes chronic or intermittent diarrhea, abdominal pain, bloating

LACTOSE INTOLERANCE

In my experience, the most common cause of abdominal discomfort, bloating, change in bowel habits, frequent loose or

diarrhea stool, and flatulence in the US non-white ethnicities (including Chinese American, African Americans, Middle Eastern Americans, immigrants from India, etc.) is lactose intolerance. These groups have genetic lactase deficiency in the intestinal brush border, and their daily symptoms will be proportional to their amount of lactose consumption. In a resource-rich country like the USA, with an abundance of inexpensive milk, dairy products in the form of different cheeses, pizza, ice cream, etc. is inviting historically dairy deprived groups to use more dairy products, because in their native land milk was scarce and culturally considered "good for your bones." Symptoms are proportional to the amount of Lactose, the milk sugar that is present in milk and dairy products, especially ice cream, soft cheeses like cottage cheese, and butter. Yogurt is significantly lactose reduced or lactose-free if sour, unless they have added lactose after initial bacterial fermentation for enhancing its taste.

Unabsorbed lactose enters the colon and is fermented by lactobacilli groups to produce lactic acid, calories, and short chain fatty acids, as well as CO_2, hydrogen and methane gases. Unfermented lactose plus fermentation products are the causes of IBS-similar symptoms. Lactose intolerance is often primary, persistent and life long, but it could be secondary to a number of GI problems, causing destruction of the brush border that wasn't present in a younger age. These symptoms will be eliminated after treatment of underlying diseases like acute gastroenteritis, small intestine bacterial overgrowth (SIBO), Celiac disease, or giardiasis. Treatments may involve drugs like olmesartan, or abdominal radiation, etc.

Diagnosis of lactase deficiency: the patient consumes 25 to 50 g of lactose, and in a breath test, measuring hydrogen in exhaled breaths, an increase beyond 20 PPM (parts per millions) within 60 to 180 minutes is considered positive. If milk is used consider that 8 ounces of milk only contains 12 g of lactose. A positive test without symptoms indicates lactose malabsorption but not intolerance. A negative test with symptoms may indicate the person being one of 20% of people who are not hydrogen excreters, and they'll have false negative tests. In this case, lactase deficiency needs to be confirmed by doing a lactose tolerance test. In this instance, patient drinks 50 g of lactose and blood sugar is measured just before drinking lactose and every 30 minutes for two hours. Any increase beyond 20 mg above the baseline is considered a positive test. The two tests have 94% sensitivity for diagnosing lactose malabsorption. False positive breath hydrogen test results can be seen in patients with SIBO.

Treatment of lactose intolerance includes reducing lactose consumption, using Lactaid milk, consuming sour yogurt without added lactose, and hard cheeses like cheddar. The amount of lactose in milk, whether whole, skim, one percent, or 2% fat is 9 to 14 g per cup. This is increased to 24 to 28 g in dry evaporated milk and 31 to 50 g in sweetened condensed milk. Whole milk has 9 to 12 g of lactose per cup, Lactaid milk could have as low as 3 grams of lactose, yogurt has 4 to 17 g of lactose per cup depending on how early the fermentation is stopped and whether they have added lactose to the yogurt in order to sweeten its taste. Ice cream, half a cup, has up to 6 g of lactose.

The patient needs to take supplemental calcium and vitamin D to prevent osteoporosis, if they find it necessary to severely restrict dairy products consumption.

Patients with severe lactose intolerance drinking a glass of milk or even using LactAid milk supplemented by lactaid pills can have symptoms because these products may not be 100% lactose-free in spite of their advertised claim, or these patients may have additional problems like milk protein allergy or fat intolerance that is causing their symptoms.

The good news is that 40% to 85% of **IBS** patients with lactose malabsorption improve on lactose-free diets. The other side of the coin is that some patients with lactose intolerance learn to use it to their advantage by drinking milk as a laxative when constipated (osmotic diarrhea).

FRUCTOSE INTOLERANCE

Fructose overload can cause **IBS** symptoms. The sweet mono-saccharide in fruits and honey is fructose. The human intestine does not have the capacity to absorb fructose. Fructose absorption is facilitated by the glucose transport system (piggy backing), which can be overloaded after large amounts of fructose intake. Therefore, fruc-tose absorption occurs mostly when taken along with glucose. Table sugar and high-fructose corn syrup have equal amounts of glucose and fructose.

Malabsorbed fructose molecules are fermented by colon bacteria and produce short chain fatty acids, hydrogen, and CO_2 similar to lactose. Healthy people absorb up to 25 grams of fructose. With 50 grams of fructose, everybody has symptoms (fructose overload). Some patients have symptoms with ingestion of as little as 3 g of fructose (fructose intolerance).

Chocolate, caramel and praline are high in fructose. They contain 30 to 40 g of fructose per hundred grams.

Increased fructose in the form of fruit juices increases useful firmicutes in stool.

Dietary sugar, especially the fructose in it, increases CRP (C Reactive Protein), a marker of low-grade inflammation. Fructose can be metabolized to uric acid. Studies have shown that high uric acid levels in blood increase asthma attacks in children.

Excess fructose intake may also be related to depression, fatty liver, and metabolic syndrome.

Reducing fructose in diet significantly benefits patients with IBS symptoms.

Eating fruits that naturally contain sorbitol and mannitol in sugar-free products can exacerbate bloating, gas and diarrhea. In addition to fructose, some fruits also contain varying amount of non-absorbable carbohydrates (see High-FODMAP list).

FOODS WITH HIGH-FODMAP CONTENTS

FERMENTABLE (OLIGO-DI-MONO) SACCHARIDES AND POLYOLS

FODMAPs are part of the family of starches that are not absorbed by the small intestine. There is no direct mechanism for fructose absorption and the intestines can be easily overloaded with it. The small intestine lacks enzymes to break down some oligosaccharides (fructans and galactans) to simple glucose, galactose and/or fructose to be able to get absorbed by the small intestinal linings. These short chain carbohydrates, however, are highly fermentable by colon bacteria producing calories, lactic acid, useful SCFAs, CO2, hydrogen and methane.

High-FODMAP foods includes:

Food high in **fructose**: apples, pears, watermelon, honey, fruit juice, dried fruits, high-fructose corn syrup, etc.

High in oligosaccharides **fructan & galactan:** wheat, rye, garlic, onion, leaks, soy, legumes, lentil, artichoke, asparagus, cabbage, broccoli, etc.

High **polyols** (sorbitol, mannitol, xylitol): stone fruits, avocado, mushroom, cauliflower, etc.

High-FODMAP foods are considered healthy and more and more people are consuming them nowadays. Once FODMAP particles reach the colon, large intestinal bacteria consume it as a source of food with byproducts of: calorie (2.5–3kcal/g), short chain fatty acid that is necessary and is the source of nutrition and health for colocytes, lactic acid and gases including large amounts of odorless hydrogen, carbon dioxide, and methane. Also depending on the amount that's consumed, small undigested food particles increase osmotic pressure which pull fluids for the bloodstream into the large intestine lumen, resulting in loose stool, diarrhea and even more mucus. The physiologic and natural end results of this phenomenon of fermentation combustion is: bloating, gas, flatulence, abdominal discomfort and pain, loose and more frequent stools with or without mucus in it. The above symptoms could be from minimal bloating to very severe, depending on the amount of FODMAP consumed (quantitative). If there are additional contributing conditions like lactose intolerance, concomitant with drinking large amounts of carbonated beverages (especially diet variety) or beer, eating and swallowing fast, swallowing too much air, slow GI transit with constipation and/or rapid small intestine transit which delivers more undigested and unabsorbed food to the large intestine. A small-framed, thin female in good shape who is constipated, has a tortuous sigmoid colon and is vegetarian is obviously more prone to feeling more severe symptoms. Other factors could include abdominal wall laxity, and the capacity for intracolonic volume expansion (while in a tight space 50 ml of gas may be too much and patients complain about bloating, a larger person with more room to spare in the colon, may be able to tolerate up to 3 liters). The presence of intraabdominal adhesions due to previous surgery, inflammation as well as psychosocial make up and level of education will play a significant role in how symptoms are perceived by the patients. For example, in India most IBS patients are well-educated, wealthy overweight males and in the US well-educated thin females. Also, there is a difference between a small-frame constipated female and a large-frame person that is not constipated, in how they perceive several bowel movements per day and how much gas they can tolerate and will consider acceptable, how much room the gases have to expand before becoming painful, how freely one can pass gas and how easily they have access to a toilet at work. Whether they have enough methane-producing bacteria in their colon to reduce hydrogen volume (methane molecule has 4 hydrogen), and enough firmicutes and lactobacilli are present in the colon microbiome (Enterotype) in order to ferment parts of or entire residual undigested food particles, whether they are a non-hydrogen excreter and how healthy their lungs are to handle extra gases are other factors. Passing gas at work, especially if malodorous, becomes unpleasant and embarrassing socially.

Most of the time, intestinal gas and flatus are a good sign and indicate that the patient is eating healthy food and the beneficial bacteria in their colon are hard at work salvaging calories, producing critical and necessary nutrients and vitamins, boosting immunity and improving the subject's mental status.

As for fiber supplements, they are hydrophilic compounds that bind water and expand. The water-soluble fiber supplements also get fermented by intestinal bacteria, and depending on quantity they may increase bloating, discomfort, and even more constipation if adequate amounts of water are not consumed along with them.

15% to 25% of IBS patients taking fiber supplements report more symptoms of bloating and distention. Only 10% of IBS patient taking fiber report improvement.

When using fiber, one has to start with a teaspoonful in a tall glass of water at night, and within 2 to 3 weeks increase gradually as tolerated to 20 to 30 grams daily.

Studies have shown that with IBS patients using all types of fibers, including methylcellulose (Citrucel), coarse bran, and psyllium (Metamucil), there is no symptom improvement. Metamucil, how-ever, helps with the ease of passage of stool. One of my fiber enthusiast colleagues, when advising IBS patients, uses the toothpaste tube analogy: If squeezed when full, the toothpaste comes out easily, but the emptier it is the harder it gets to squeeze it out.[1]

FOOD INTOLERANCE

Food intolerances may be related to pharmacologic agents in the food, like caffeine (coffee), theobromine (tea and chocolate), histamine and histamine-like compounds (berries, wine, fish, and sauerkraut), Tryptamine (tomatoes and plum), tyramine (cheese and

---

1   For the list of low FODMAP foods please see:
    www.GERD-IBS.com/IBS/FODMAP diet

pickled fish), serotonin (banana and tomato), phenylethylamine (chocolate), solamine (potatoes), alcohol, flavoring and preservatives (MSG and sodium sulfite).

Obviously, given the right setting the quantity of foods ingested correlates with severity of symptoms.

FOOD ALLERGY

Up to 20% of adults in the general population report recurrent adverse reactions to a specific food or food groups, and more than half of them have IBS symptoms. Most are examples of food intolerance which are non-immunologic and non-allergic reactions to food. They can be due to a host of disorders, including GERD, metabolic disease, toxin mediated, GI infections, digestive enzyme deficiency, anatomic and neurological abnormalities and other processes.

The true food allergy that is IgE mediated does not typically present with IBS-type symptoms.

IgE-mediated food allergy is a medical emergency and it will only be mentioned here due to its significance. In rare cases, exposure to minute amounts of these foods may produce nausea, severe abdominal cramps partly relieved by bowel movements (getting rid of allergen), bloating and diarrhea. It could be mistaken as IBS by a novice.

Up to 5% of adults have this IgE type of food allergy, which is due to allergen-induced sudden widespread activation of mast cells and basophils releasing chemicals.

15% of patients first diagnosed with this kind of food allergy are adult, and symptoms peak in their 30s, but may first appear as late as their mid-80s. Food allergy symptoms includes: pruritus, urticaria (hives), flushing, swelling of the lips, face or throat, nausea, vomiting, abdominal cramps, diarrhea, wheezing, light-headedness, syncope, and hypotension within five to 20 minutes of ingestion of the offending food.

Acute urticaria is the most common early symptom. Anaphylaxis is a potentially life-threatening allergic reaction that can occur within seconds or minutes of exposure to an allergen, like peanuts.

Factors that can cause more severe food-related allergic reactions and anaphylaxis in these patients include: concomitant asthma, use of agents that increase intestinal permeability like alcoholics beverages, aspirin, NSAIDs, exertion, stress, concomitant viral illness, lack of sleep and menstruation. Anti-hypertension medications like ACE inhibitors and beta-blockers prevent blood pressure from going up when they become hypotensive and need an epinephrine injection to save their life.

Two unusual presentations worth mentioning include delayed allergy to red meat 3 to 6 hours after ingestion (usually late night or after midnight after dining out at a steak house, waking up with severe allergic symptoms), and food dependent exercise-induced anaphylaxis.

In the United States, fish/seafood and peanuts/tree nuts are the two food group that causes most IgE-mediated food allergies.

Rarely, a patient will have food allergies that present within 10 to 30 minutes of being exposed to the offending agent, usually in restaurants.

I have seen several patients with a garlic allergy. With negligible amounts of garlic in their food in spite of notifying the restaurant's chef and taking precautions, they'll develop severe abdominal cramping, nausea, and diarrhea within 5–20 minutes of being exposed to garlic in their meal. This will abate after several diarrheal movements, but abdominal discomfort may last from a couple of hours to a couple of days. This garlic allergy prevalence is increasing, and unfortunately garlic has penetrated American cuisine as much as gluten and peanuts.

Also, patients who are allergic to aspirin and NSAIDs may have IBS symptoms when ingesting high-salicylate foods like avocado, black berry, guava, tomato, etc. I have seen similar cases of allergies to walnut, strawberry, chicken, eggplant and thyme with similar symptoms to garlic allergy. Some patients may have a food allergy related to latex contamination from preparation or packaging.

Patients with a true food allergy must see and be evaluated by an allergist for diagnosis and treatment, avoid the allergen, carry an epinephrine autoinjector, and in severe cases, have a wrist band indicating their condition and the location of epinephrin if in their possession or the emergent need for it in case of anaphylaxis.

Food allergy testing is typically done by a skin test, in vitro testing, and food challenges. Studies have shown that in children two years and older with IgE-mediated food allergy, egg, milk, peanuts, tree nuts and fish are the most common foods allergens.

In some patients with IBS, there have been some blood tests directed toward multiple potential allergens to look for specific food protein IgG antibody in their blood. Elimination of the responsible food as identified by having an IgG antibody toward that food antigen has been proposed, but the relationship with symptom improvement is not clear. Methods used in evaluating food allergies (for example, the skin prick test, RAST testing, and atopy patch testing) have not been well standardized. Testing for food specific immunoglobulin G and IgG4 yields multiple positive test results and may represent normal immune responses to foods.

Eosinophilic esophagitis and food protein-induced enterocolitis are non-IgE-mediated conditions.

CELIAC SPRUE (GLUTEN ALLERGY) AND GLUTEN SENSITIVITY

It is estimated that about three million Americans have celia sprue. In US 5% of patient with IBS diagnosis have celiac disease.

Celiac is an autoimmune disease in patients who are allergic to a group of energy-storing proteins called prolamins. They include gliadin in wheat, secalins in rye, and hordeins in barley.

In genetically susceptible patients, with HLA-DQ 2 & DQ8, exposure to these proteins will cause damage to the inner lining of the small intestine, resulting in a combination of maldigestion of disaccharides like lactose and malabsorption of already digested nutritional materials ready to enter blood stream.

Signs and symptoms depend on the degree of damage to enterocytes, and the resulting nutritional deficiencies.

Clinically, 77% of patients with celiac sprue have abdominal pain, 73% report gas and bloating, 52% experience diarrhea, 7% have constipation and 24% alternate between diarrhea and constipation.

Iron deficiency anemia, weight loss, delayed puberty, osteoporosis, skin rash (dermatitis herpetiformis), type one diabetes mellitus, autoimmune thyroiditis, Down's syndrome, and infertility are some other health-related conditions caused by, or more often associated with, celiac disease.

Diagnosis of celiac is confirmed by positive blood test for TTG Ab, IgA type, intraepithelial lymphocytosis on duodenal biopsy, and response to a gluten-free diet (clinical improvement, normalization of both TTG ab and duodenal biopsy).

However, an abnormal biopsy typical of celiac sprue (that is duodenal lymphocytosis and villous atrophy), even though diagnostic for celiac, is non-specific and can be seen with multiple conditions including: non-gluten protein allergy (chicken, cow milk, eggs, fish, rice, and soy), H. pylori infection, SIBO and blind loop syndrome, NSAIDs use, dermatitis herpetiformis, eosinophilic enteritis, IBD, giardiasis, SB lymphoma, post gastroenteritis, tropical sprue, Zollinger Ellison syndrome, autoimmune enteritis, SLE, type 1 diabetes mellitus, microscopic colitis, and the use of various medications. Needless to say, all of the aforementioned conditions are capable of producing IBS type symptoms.

GLUTEN SENSITIVITY

There is a group of patients that report bloating and abdominal discomfort when eating food containing gluten. In some of these patients, anti-gliadin IgG antibody may be positive, and they are positive for permissing HLADQ2/&DQ8. These patients are suffering from latent celiac disease.

Some gluten sensitive patients with a family history of celiac and negative comprehensive celiac panel blood test results report benefiting from gluten restriction in relieving bloating, abdominal discomfort, diarrhea or constipation, skin rash and fatigue. They insist on staying on expensive gluten-free diets. These patients are often young to middle-aged females, thin, highly educated, and economically able society members. It's possible that reducing carbohydrates in the diet in order to eliminate gluten makes them feel better (less FODMAP). SIBO, rapid intestinal transit time or leaky-gut syndrome cause symptoms that respond to gluten restriction. One needs to rule out the aforementioned conditions, and if necessary perform a 5 hour urine lactulose-mannitol test to see if leaky gut symptoms are present (fatigue, skin rash, cloudy mental status & IBS symptoms).

In patients who have been on a gluten-free diet for several months, the TTG Ab blood test and small bowel biopsy may be normal even if they have celiac sprue. Other than putting them back on a gluten-containing diet (usually not recommended) and repeating the TTG Ab and duodenal biopsy, the only other test that may help is to determine if they are HLA-DQ 2 &DQ8 positive. If so, they may have celiac sprue, but if blood tests are negative for HLADQ2 & DQ8, then there's no chance that they have celiac sprue.

In patients with IgA deficiency, a TTG ab IgA Test may present a false negative. That's why, when suspicious, in addition to TTGab IgA, serum IgA level is checked to make sure we are not dealing with IgA deficiency. In these instances Gliadin Ab IgG, HLA subtyping plus duodenal biopsy are helpful diagnostic tests.

As for gluten-free diets, in addition to obvious sources of gluten, there are hidden gluten-containing foods. For example, even ketchup, instant coffee and frozen custard may have gluten. So, it's important to read all the commercially prepared food and additive ingredients, because celiac is an autoimmune disease and minimal exposure to gluten can trigger reactivation of allergy and autoimmune cascade. Also, consult a dietitian with expertise in celiac with the latest knowledge in gluten-free foods and additives.

SMALL INTESTINAL BACTERIAL OVERGROWTH (SIBO)

There are about 10,000 bacteria in each gram of contents of small bowel, as compared to 10 billion bacteria in a gram of stool, therefore small bowel is relatively sterile. SIBO occurs because of slow transit and/or stagnation of small intestinal contents locally or diffusely, and there are more than a million bacteria per gram of contents.

Some medical conditions responsible for SIBO are diabetic visceral neuropathy, small bowel diverticulosis, obesity surgery like gastric and intestinal bypass (blind loop), localized narrowing from adhesions, enteritis like Crohn's, systemic sclerosis, chronic intestinal pseudo obstruction, chronic pancreatitis, and a lack of gastric acid to kill bacteria passing thru the stomach into the small intestine and chronic use of medications like PPIs and NSAIDs. However, 90% of cases of SIBO are related to intestinal motility disorders and chronic pancreatitis.

SIBO is not an infection but an overgrowth of normal colon (large bowel) type of bacteria in the wrong place (small bowel). Bacteria are mostly coliforms like bifidobacteria and lactobacilli. Abundances of bacteria in SB function like bacteria in the colon, and when exposed to semi-digested and unabsorbed food they ferment what is fermentable and produce calories, hydrogen, CO_2, and rarely methane (only if methane-producing bacteria are present too).

Patients with SIBO may have elevated folate and vitamin K levels that are produced by these bacteria, and low B12 used by bacteria. Too much bacteria in the small bowel additionally causes maldigestion and malabsorption due to damaging enterocyte villi and altering motility, "adding injury to insult."

Symptoms includes bloating, postprandial abdominal discomfort that starts a couple of hours after eating, and diarrhea, similar to IBS. Diarrhea is a mixture of loose acidic diarrhea from carbohydrate fermentation and fatty foul smelling due to fat malabsorption. Occasionally a patient will present with the only chief complaint being weight loss. Bacteria also damage bile acids (deconjugation) to cause fat malabsorption with associated fat soluble vitamin deficiency, producing foul-smelling fatty stools similar to chronic pancreatitis.

In the US, 4% of IBS patients are found to have SIBO. Additionally, in 75% of IBS patients bloating and abdominal discomfort improves with a short course of antibiotics like Rifaximin and Neomycin. This is most likely because these antibiotics significantly reduce the number of fermenting bacteria like lactobacilli and bifidobacteria in the colon too, hence improvement regardless of whether patient has SIBO or not.

SIBO is diagnosed by doing a lactulose breath test in which the patient drinks a certain amount of lactulose (indigestible but fermentable disaccharide) and hydrogen is measured in breath. A positive test result shows an increase of 20 ppm hydrogen in exhaled breath 90 minutes after swallowing lactulose. However, if the patient has taken antibiotics within a month before the test it could be false negative. Also, a patient who has delayed gastric emptying it could produce a false negative. Also, a patient with rapid small bowel transit time it may show a false positive because unabsorbed lactulose will reach colon bacteria where fermentation occurs. Using glucose to do a breath test is more accurate because glucose gets completely absorbed in the small intestine, and unlike lactulose that does not get absorbed and needs to have bacteria for fermentation (which can only occur if fermicutes are present), glucose is absorbed without the need for bacteria and does not need to be fermented and won't produce Hydrogen, unless it is exposed to bacteria before it has a chance for normal absorption. A glucose breath test is more specific for proximal small intestine SIBO. Cultures of small bowel contents taken to look for SIBO are not practical because intubation is required to obtain small intestinal contents. In addition, a strict anaerobic environment is required during collection and culture, a rather difficult task.

Treatment of SIBO involves taking Rifaximin (Xifaxan) 550 mg by mouth three times a day for two weeks.

If a breath test reveals additional methane-producing bacteria, it is necessary to add neomycin 500 mg twice a day for 10 to 14 days. Because of insurance issues, Rifaximin may not be covered due to expense. Other antibiotics like Ciprofloxacin, Bactrim, metronidazole, tetracycline, and Augmentin are effective and may be substituted.

If there are pathological reasons for recurring SIBO that can't be corrected easily, the patient may require further treatments when symptoms recur. Additional treatments may take place at different intervals, from monthly to every 3 to 6 months of full course, or just one week a month. The patient may even be prescribed a low-dose antibiotic daily. These intervals will depend on the cause, frequency and severity of symptoms.

Both Rifaximin and Neomycin are GI antibiotics, and very little is systematically absorbed, so they are without significant side effects if used for a short period of time.

Of interest is one study that showed 37% of patients with non-alcoholic fatty liver disease (NAFLD) have E. Coli (proteobacter) predominant SIBO, speculating that SIBO may be causing leaky gut, allowing bacterial toxin absorption and liver injury.

BILE ACID DIARRHEA

Bile acids are produced and conjugated in the liver (0.2–0.6g/day), stored and concentrated in the gallbladder. Then a meal is transferred from the gall bladder to the small intestine in order to participate in digestion and absorption of fat.

97% of bile acid is reabsorbed by the terminal ileum (enterohepatic circulation), and small amounts are lost to the colon (0.2–0.6g/ day in health). Biliary secretions = pool x cycle (pool 3 g, cycles occurs 4–12 times/day), hence there are 12–36 g of bile secreted and absorbed daily.

In chronic inflammatory liver disease and bile duct or pancreatic cancer there is reduced availability of bile (blockage) for normal absorption of dietary fat.

Fat malabsorption causes fatty foul smelling, clay colored diarrheal stool. Chemically changed bile acids by bacteria (deconjugation) in SIBO, and Crohn's disease of terminal ileum or surgically removed terminal ileum, causes the delivery of excess unabsorbed bile acid into the colon.

In the large intestine, bile acid acts like a strong laxative (increases secretion and enhances motility), plus it damages the mucus layer (chenodeoxycholic acid & deoxycholic acid). Dietary emulsifiers present in margarine and some baby formula also act like bile acids. Bile acid-induced diarrhea is a relatively common cause of chronic IBS-D, It may be **primary** due to excess bile acid production by the liver, idiopathic bile acid malabsorption in terminal ileum, and rapid intestinal transit, or **secondary** to ileal disease or resection of terminal ileum resulting in reduced absorptive surface in terminal ileum, causing excess delivery of bile to the colon.

Diarrhea due to excess bile acid delivered to the colon in extreme cases is sudden in onset, starting with severe lower abdominal cramps and urgency followed by explosive yellowish watery diarrhea that, if not relieved, may cause fecal incontinence. Severity of symptoms is dose dependent and may change from one day to another.

Bile acid diarrhea is seen in 10% of patients after gall bladder surgery, because bile is continuously moving from the liver into the gut and storage place is gone now. Diarrhea usually resolves within 2 to 3 months; however, in 3% of patients it will continue for the rest of their life. Perhaps to begin with, they are genetically high-bile-acid producers in the liver or poor reabsorbers in terminal ileum.

For treatment, bile acid binding resin cholestyramine (Questran) powder works like magic. Within a few days those episodes of severe crampy, watery bowel movements and fecal incontinence resolve. The amount required for each patient is different, from 4 g to 12 g daily. As they become more stable, 1–2 Colestipol tablets a day may suffice in order to maintain normal bowel movements.

In patients with intractable bile acid diarrhea not responding or not willing to take more than 2 packets of Questran daily, I have added Farnesoid X receptor agonist Obethicolic acid (Ocaliva 5–10 mg tablets). Obethicolic acid reduces bile acid synthesis in the liver and results in a beneficial synergistic effect with cholestyramine powder that binds them. Ocaliva is contraindicated in patients with liver cirrhosis.

There are a group of patients with IBS symptoms similar to bile acid diarrhea but with no history of gallbladder removal and/ or Ileal resection (primary bile acid diarrhea). These people may have excess bile acid production, genetic reduced absorption, rapid small bowel transit not giving ileum enough time for normal absorption or SIBO. Treating them with cholestyramine powder will resolve their IBS symptoms as well.

Cholestyramine taste is not pleasant, patients say it's like drinking sand. It doesn't get absorbed, it binds cholesterol and brings serum cholesterol down too. In fact, before the Statin era, it was the main medication for treatment of hypercholesterolemia. It also binds other medications, making them less available to the body. I tell patients to dissolve it in orange juice, take it within 2–4 hours of other meds, and on a full stomach to prevent nausea (usually after lunch or after dinner if taking multiple meds otherwise after breakfast).

A colestipol tablet is large, containing one gram of Cholestyramine. Some patients find it easier to take than the powder. I recommend 1–2 daily empirically in some IBS patients when clinical scenarios suggest possible bile-induced IBS.

Some studies suggest that up to 30% of IBS-D may be secondary to bile acid malabsorption, 40% dietary intolerance and 20% SIBO.

Increased levels of fecal bile acids have been found in patients with IBS-D as well as functional diarrhea.[2]

LEAKY GUT

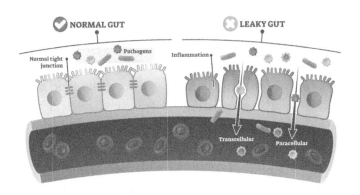

Leaky gut is present when intestinal defense barriers become defective and allow entry of microbes or large molecules into the body when otherwise it would not be possible.

The intestinal barrier includes a surface mucus layer preventing bacterial adhesion by viscosity, secretion of IgA and defensins, epithelial cells connected at the tight junction by junctional complex which have the ability to transport luminal content and react to noxious stimuli by secretion of chloride and antimicrobial peptides, and the lamina propria with innate and acquired immune cells secreting immune globulins and cytokines.

Epithelial permeability results from increased paracellular transport due to damaged tight junction, apoptosis (programmed cell death), erosions and ulcers, as well as trans-cellular permeability from cell damage and sickness.

---

2   Walters, J. R., Johnston, I. M., Nolan, J. D., Vassie, C., Pruzanski, M. E., & Shapiro, D. A. (2015). The response of patients with bile acid diarrhoea to the farnesoid X receptor agonist obeticholic acid. *Aliment Pharmacol Ther*, *41*(1), 54–64. https://doi.org/10.1111/apt.12999

Leaky gut allows entrance of undesirable materials like antigens, large foreign molecules via apoptosis leaks, bacteria and macromolecules via erosions and ulcers and sick epithelial cells (transcytosis). Symptoms includes mid to lower abdominal discomfort, bloating, diarrhea or constipation, and in some cases cloudy mental status, extreme fatigue and even skin rash.

Leaky gut is also thought to cause multiple food allergies and intolerances, joint pain, different autoimmune diseases, chronic fatigue syndrome, fibromyalgia, skin rash, fatty liver, NASH, and so on.

Patients who have problems (intolerance or allergy) with a variety of foods may be suffering from leaky gut.

Gluten, sugar and milk may increase leaky gut. Fermented foods like kimchi, sauerkraut, yogurt, kefir, and pickles may help repair leaky gut.

Supplements like L. glutamine, vitamin D, zinc, omega-3 fatty acids in fish oil and good bacteria in probiotics may also help repair leaky gut.

Endurance exercises, marathon running, NSAIDs, alcohol use, SIBO with toxin producing E Coli, deficient secretory IgA, Ehler Donlos syndrome, HIV, Crohn's, autoimmune enteritis, trauma, endotoxinemia, intestinal infection, excess bile acids, dietary emulsifiers and food allergens may increase intestinal permeability causing or exacerbating IBS symptoms.

Diagnosis of Leaky Gut is established by the lactulose-mannitol (LM) test. Patients consume a certain amount of lactulose (disaccharide with large size) and mannitol (monosaccharides with small size). Urine is collected for 5 hours and if leaky gut is present there will be lactulose in the urine. The amount of lactulose plus lactulose mannitol ratio will determine how severe and extensive the leaky gut is.

Treatment includes addressing or removing the offending cause, a low-FODMAP diet, the reduction or elimination of gluten from diet, pre-biotics and probiotics like Kefir or yogurt to produce desirable butyrate, zinc, glutamine, fish oil and if bile acid is suspected cholestyramine, to repair the leaks.

Dicyclomine may be used for pain and cramps if present.[3]

POST GASTROENTERITIS IBS

Symptoms of bloating, abdominal discomfort, and diarrhea alternating with constipation can last up to eight years after an episode of acute bacterial gastroenteritis. In these patients there is a low-grade inflammation in the small intestine and colon mucosa, plus changes in gut microflora.

Treatments that have been tried include trials of anti-inflammatory NSAIDs and 5-ASA (Mesalamin), poorly absorbed antibiotics like Rifaximin and Neomycin to target stasis bacteria, and positively changing gut flora with prebiotics and probiotics.

Pre-biotics like bran and inulin promote growth of commensal bacteria like lactobacilli and bifidobacteria throughout the colon. Commercially available symbiotics are combinations of probiotic and prebiotic with synergic effect like: bifidobacterium plus Fructo-oligosaccharide, galacto-oligosaccharides, lactobacillus rhamnosuss, and lactobacillus GG plus inulin. However, evidence remains unconvincing for benefits of 5-ASA and probiotics in treating IBS symptoms.

Chronic GI infection with Giardia, Ameba, Blastocystis Hominis and Candida Albicans can mimic IBS symptoms.

MICROSCOPIC COLITIS

Microscopic colitis is the cause of up to 5% of patients presenting as IBS diarrhea.

Patients are usually middle-aged females complaining of severe watery diarrhea, 7–15 times daily including diarrhea at night with occasional fecal incontinence. They have minimal cramps (difference with bile-induced diarrhea), and there's no blood in the stools.

---

3   Camilleri, M. (2019). Leaky gut: mechanisms, measurement and clinical implications in humans. *Gut*, *68*(8), 1516–1526.
    https://doi.org/10.1136/gutjnl-2019–318427

Work up for Chronic watery Diarrhea is negative including Celiac serology. Colonoscopy is normal but biopsy shows lymphocytic and/or collagenous colitis.

It responds to a locality active GI steroid called budesonide (Entecort 3 mg tablet), beginning with 9 mg after breakfast daily.

Usually few weeks of treatment with tapering the dose will suffice but some patient may need long-term low-dose (3mg) maintenance treatment.

On colonoscopy colon lining looks normal and unless multiple biopsies are taken from the entire colon diagnosis may be missed.

Flexible sigmoidoscopy and multiple biopsies is diagnostic in 90% of cases. Rectal biopsy is not enough and could be false negative, but colonoscopy with multiple biopsies from different segments of colon specially cecum and ascending colon is 100% positive because disease activity is more severe in proximal colon.

Medication that is known to cause microscopic colitis includes aspirin, NSAIDs, proton pump inhibitors especially lansoprazole, Statins used for high cholesterol, sertraline, ticlopidine, acarbose, novel anti-cancer medication keytruda, cigarette smoking.

Up to one third of patients with celiac sprue on colon bx have lymphocytic colitis.

BRAINARD DIARRHEA

Brainard diarrhea is an epidemic of watery (secretory) diarrhea of unknown etiology.

Small bowel biopsy shows patchy lymphocytic infiltrate. It can last up to three years before spontaneous resolution.

It is speculated that it may be due to a not yet identified bacteria or virus.

CHRONIC DIARRHEA DUE TO CANDIDA ALBICANS

Very rarely in some patients with IBS symptoms, the only abnormal finding may be a large number of candida albicans (yeast that causes thrush in children and candida esophagitis in immunocompromised adults) in stool or small bowel aspirates. There is a favorable response to anti-fungal treatment.

Good bacteria in the GI tract are important in digesting starches, fibers, and some sugars. Imbalance of bacteria and overgrowth of candida can cause digestive issues like constipation, diarrhea, nausea, gas, bloating, and cramps. Factors that can lead to overgrowth of candida in the GI tract includes taking long-term steroids inhalers for asthma and COPD, strong antibiotics, eating a diet. high in sugar and refined carbohydrates, high alcohol intake, weakened immune system, oral contraceptives, diabetes mellitus, and high stress level. Treatment with fluconazole is curative.

IBS & CONSTIPATION

In the US 63 million people admit to chronic constipation. Constipation is defined as less than 3 bowel movements per week. Stool is hard and lumpy. Constipation is more prevalent in women.

Several times daily after meals, especially after breakfast, the stomach communicate to the colon via a gastrocolic reflex (nerve, muscle, hormones) that food will be coming and to start emptying some stool to make room for the coming residues. Propulsive movements from the proximal colon to the rectum pushes colon contents forward by squeezing it, and if everything works the way it should, we voluntarily help ourself when the feeling comes and the time is right by relaxing anal sphincters and pelvic floor muscles, and squeeze the abdominal wall to accomplish defecation.

Under ideal situations the colon has enough stool in it that is moist, large and easy to move because it is covered with mucus as a lubricant. The colon also needs to have a healthy nervous system, musculature tone, contents and the right environment to respond properly. Any deficiency in this complex process, including not responding to "Mother Nature" when she calls can end up causing constipation. Not drinking enough water, not taking in enough roughage and not paying attention after breakfast, allowing for stool to accumulate, harden and dilate the colon, will slowly but surely cause system derangement, and worsening of constipation.

I can't put it any better than what one of my colleagues (AP) has so famously come up with, the "tooth paste tube analogy". When it's full slight pressure is enough to push out toothpaste, when relatively. empty you need to squeeze it harder, even fold it to get a small amount of toothpaste out.

Most constipation is related to or starts with no obvious reason except minor issues like not enough fiber in the diet, sedentary life style, not enough water intake and not being able to go when gastro-colic peristalsis is in motion. This is called functional constipation, and is common especially amongst women. The other 11% is due to slow transit, 13% dyssynergic defecation due to pelvis floor problems and 5% combination of slow transit and dyssynergic defecation.

Metabolic problems like diabetes, hypothyroidism, hypercalcemia, hypokalemia and hypomagnesimia, as well as multiple medications like calcium channel blockers, anticholinergics, antidepressants, antipsychotics, anxiolytics, iron supplements, opiates, sucralfate, aluminum containing antacids without MOM, diuretics, etc. also causes constipation.

A constipated patient has the same issues with poorly absorbed carbohydrates, lactose, fructose etc., that a normal person has, only worse. These issues include bloating, gas, irregular bowel movements, abdominal pain and cramps depending on the degree of constipation and amount of indigestible food that was consumed. The byproduct of it is now locked in behind stool and not able to easily pass. These patients with constipation may have days with diarrhea depending on their diet, hence the term **IBS-Mix (IBS-M)**.

EVALUATION OF IBS PATIENTS IN THE CLINIC

Reason for visit: bloating, abdominal discomfort, change in bowel habits, frequent bowel movements, constipation, changing stool form, abdominal distention. Which one is the main reason for the visit?

History of present illness: after listening to the chief complaint, this is the most important part of the visit, and if done right often the physician will have a pretty good idea that what is going on or what direction evaluation should be taken.

When did symptoms **start**? what is the **duration**? Is it getting worse? What are **bowel movements** like (if diarrhea is present, is it watery, small but frequent with mucus, contain gross blood, does it float, is it malodorous, frothy, is there a large volume, is it present even when fasting)? Has there been any **change in diet**? Is the type of diet mostly meat and fat, mostly fruits and vegetables, or vegetarian? What is the time of diet change and it's relation with symptoms? How is the patient's **psychosocial life**, any job changes or restrictions? Where is the pain, how often does it occur, how serious is it? What is the relation with bowel movements, before, during or after? Is there any food intolerance or allergy? What **medications** is the patient taking, are there any new meds or recent changes in meds? Has the patient undergone any **surgery** like gall bladder removal, gastric bypass or surgery for release of intraabdominal adhesions? Is there gynecological or gastrointestinal cancer present, or diverticulitis? Any **antibiotic** use within the last 6 month. Any recent use of **fiber** supplements, any **travel** abroad, any well water drinking or camping in the woods? What is the **dairy** intake (quantity and type of milk and cheeses)? What is the intake of soda, **diet foods and drinks,** coffee, alcohol, chocolate? Is there a past history of acute gastroenteritis, especially if hospitalization was required? What is the use and pattern of alcoholic beverages? Is there any **food intolerance or allergy, concomitant** medical problems like DM, hypo or hyperthyroidism, hypertension, and autoimmune problems, or radiation to abdomen? What are the activity and stress levels? Is the patient a marathon runner? Is the patient taking **over the counter** meds and supplements like herbal tea, magnesium supplements, antacids, laxatives, anti-diarrhea medications, etc?

Review of systems: fever, abdominal pain, pain location and grade, weight loss, anorexia, change in appetite, nausea and vomiting, blood in the stool, nocturnal bowel movements. Is diarrhea present when fasting, any fat or blood in it or visible mucus? Finally, past evaluation, if any, for the same problem (results, any diet or medication trial).

Medication: especially ask about metformin and its daily dose, proton pump inhibitors (especially Lansoprazole) and daily dose, antacids (type and amount), prokinetics, antidepressanst, trulicity, acarbose, olmesartan, narcotics, anticholinergics, and NSAIDs. Make sure to name them, including generics and over the counter names. Ask about steroids, statins, and cigarette smoking.

Allergies to meds, foods, and the type of allergic reaction.

Past history of any intraabdominal surgery for: removal of gall bladder (bile-induced diarrhea), hiatal hernia repair (gas-bloat), gastric bypass (dumping), small bowel obstruction requiring hospitalization, surgical or medical management (SIBO), short bowel, adhesions.

Family history of celiac, IBS, IBD, gi cancer, lactose intolerance, etc.

Physical exam: abdominal flat, tenderness location if present, palpable mass, bowel sounds hyper or hypo active, ascites, hepatomegaly.

A rectal exam is a must when evaluating a patient with IBS. Are there note-worthy hemorrhoids (external or internal)? What are their grade? Check for fistula, fissure, stricture, painful digital exam, sphincter tone, observation of external anal sphincter and pelvic floor movements in response to bearing down. Is there anorectal prolapse? Examine fecal impaction, and stools (hard, soft, liquids, mucus, gross blood or occult blood positive, palpable mass).

Impression:

Several scenarios will emerge from the visit:

1- positive alarm symptoms and signs, needs urgent evaluation. Not part of this discussion.

2- patient with severe watery diarrhea and previously negative complete work up, poorly responsive to usual dose of anti-diarrhea medications.

A- if middle-aged female or older male on multiple meds, 5–15 bowel movements daily including nocturnal bowel movements, may be associated with fecal incontinence. This patient most likely has microscopic colitis (lymphocytic or collagenous). Needs flexible sigmoidoscopy or colonoscopy with multiple biopsies for diagnosis.

When confirmed will respond very nicely to stopping offending medications and oral Budesonide if necessary.

B- patient with frequent episodes of sudden onset abdominal cramps, urgency and diarrhea, with rare fecal incontinence. Usually knows all the public bathrooms in the mall or when traveling, may be even wearing a diaper. This patient diarrhea is due to excess bile acid reaching the colon and mostly after Gall bladder surgery, less often terminal ileum resection due to Crohn's. This pattern of IBS is due to bile acids and it could also be seen to a lesser extent in patients with SIBO and also overproduction of bile in the liver.

Treatment of bile acid-induced diarrhea is with binding resin cholestyramine powder. The starting dose is 4 grams daily but occasionally up to 16 G may be required.

3- the most common presentation is abdominal bloating and distention, abdominal discomfort and pain, abnormally shaped stools with irregular bowel movements from several small bowel movements daily to mucusy mushy stools, a feeling of urgency and incomplete emptying. These symptoms are often daily but it need not be.

Here etiology is often the diet and is mostly carbohydrate related, from carbohydrate overload causing malabsorption, to lactose intolerance, fructose intolerance, high-FODMAP food, too much dairy products, diet candies, and other causes of malabsorption and maldigestion.

Going over daily dietary habits, fluids intake, fruit and fruit juices, V8 juice, shakes, frappes, juicing different fruits and vegetables, coffee both regular and decaf, carbonated beverages regular or sugar-free, and medications interfering with carbohydrates absorption may result in good information and reveal the reason/s for symptoms.

Here eliminating high-FODMAP fruits and vegetables, sugar-free/ sugar substitute/ diet products (sorbitol, mannitol, reducing dairy and gluten, coffee, carbonated beverages regular or sugar-free, and fiber supplements of any kind, stopping or reducing metformin, acarbose, trulicity, PPIs and NSAIDs may be helpful.

It is important to remember that unless all offending factors are eliminated, the patient may continue to have less intense IBS symptoms. It may be more practical to restrict foods in stages like wheat, eggs, dairy, high-salicylate food, fiber supplements, sugar and gluten first, and if flatus is the main issue beans, onion, celery, carrot, raisin, apricot, prune, Brussel sprouts, wheat germ, pretzels, V8 juice and bagels should be restricted. If there is no improvement go lactose-free, gluten-free with a strict low-FODMAP diet.

Labs: CBC, comprehensive metabolic profile, CRP, sec rate, TTG ab, stool for Fecal occult blood test, stool lactoferrin or calprotectin if positive indicates inflammation and possible IBD not IBS, and O&P if diarrhea present.

Patients may require a lactose tolerance or lactose breath test to look for lactase deficiency. In some patients with this regimen symptoms improves, but if bloating or distention continues without being constipated, SIBO needs to be considered and ruled out with a lactulose breath test, especially if predisposing factors exist. In addition to SIBO, a significant number of patients with IBS-D and bloating may benefit from a course of antibiotics by reducing bacterial volume and fermentation process without much of a diet change, and bile acid binding resin Questran if there is any suggestion of excess bile delivery to the large intestine.

If IBS symptoms continue, further evaluation of cause as described in differential diagnosis should be considered. If nothing is found then real IBS may be a possibility.

HIGH FODMAP (FRUITS AND VEGETABLES)

If you are suffering from on and off bloating, abdominal distention, gas, abdominal discomfort, diarrhea, irregular bowel habits, and flatulence because of eating several portions of "healthy" fruits and vegetables high in FODMAP, it means that you have a healthy colon microbiome with plenty of good "probiotic" bacteria in it, that efficiently extracts calories, very useful short chain fatty acids like butyrate, etc. and as a result more frequent bowel movements and gas. In your case it seems to be too much of a good thing and you are overdoing it, because it gives you trouble and interferes with quality of life. You need to correct baseline constipation if present because it will make symptoms worse, and use as little non digestible but fermentable foods (FODMAP) as possible in relation to your ability to tolerate gas. Using commercial products like **Lactaid** pills if lactose intolerant and Lactaid milk or almond milk as a substitute, **Beano, gas free soak,** drops when using beans and legumes, **Sucraid** drops for IBS patients with congenital sucrase-isomaltase deficiency, **gluten cutters** for gluten use, **activated charcoal** with chlorophyll tablets, **Gas-X** etc. may help to make symptom more tolerable.

Beans, cabbage, Brussel sprouts, broccoli and cauliflower are especially high in FODMAP. Excess use of soluble fibers present in oats, bran, barley, nuts, seeds, beans, lentils, peas and some fruits and vegetables can increase IBS symptoms.

Honey, coffee, carbonated beverages, alcohol, fruit juices, energy drinks and chocolate are amongst the foods often forgotten or ignored when evaluating IBS patients.

The following is a guide for foods high in FODMAP to avoid, and alternative low-FODMAP fruits and vegetables.

Application of additional fecal biomarkers when evaluating complicated IBS patients depending on your clinical suspicions includes:

Pancreatic elastase, fecal bile acids, eosinophil protein X , occult blood, H pylori Ag, C.difficile assay, parasites such as blastocystis hominid, giardia lamblia, stool Culture for quantitating beneficial bacteria, and real time PCR analysis of 12 enteric pathogens in post infectious IBS-D.[4]

---

4 Goepp J, Fowler E, McBride T, Landis D. *Frequency of Abnormal Fecal Biomarkers in Irritable Bowel Syndrome.* Global Advances in Health and Medicine Journal, May 2014, v 3, N 3, pages 9-15

HIGH-FODMAP FOODS

1. High in Fructose

The capacity at which fructose is absorbed ranges from 15–50 g per day with greatest absorption occurring when glucose and fructose are administered in equal amounts.

Apples, pears, watermelon, honey, fruit juices, dried fruits, high-fructose corn syrup, figs, plums, dates, papaya, commercial foods and soft drinks with added high-fructose corn syrup.

Studies have shown that fructose and sorbitol ingested together cause worsening of IBS symptoms.

2. High in Polyols

Stone fruits, plums, cherries, avocados, mushrooms, cauliflower, sugar alcohols (sorbitol, mannitol, xylitol, isomalto), apples, pears, peaches and prunes are high in sorbitol. Sugar-free desserts, cookies, syrup and gums have sorbitol as sweetener. Berries have xylitol.

After ingestion of 12.5 g of lactulose, up to eight times as much gas production is observed in normal individuals.

Most artificial sweeteners contain polyols such as mannitol, xylitol or sorbitol. Substances such as toothpaste, mints, sugar-free gum, and many liquid cough and cold syrups and pain reliever preparations have polyols. Patients with small bowel bacterial overgrowth appear to be even more sensitive to foods containing polyols.

3. High in Fructans and galactans

Soluble fiber is found in starches and is the chemical bond that joins its individual sugar units, and there is no enzyme in the human digestive tract to digest it.

High Fructans and galactans are present in wheat, rye, garlic, onion, artichoke, asparagus, soy, leeks, legume beans, peas, lentils, cabbage, Brussel sprouts, broccoli, chicory root, tequila that is made from fermentation of lanolin, soluble fibers inulin and maltodextrin, polydextrose made from glucose plus sorbitol added as sweetness to some food and drinks, diet soda, diet candies, and sweetened sugar-free foods and beverages.

Inulin is a polysaccharide, and belongs to a class of soluble fiber known as fructans. It is found in roots and rhizomes as a means of storing energy. It's a non-digestible carbohydrate that feels like fat and is chewy, and it has many applications in the food industry. Garlic bulb has a lot of inulin.

Sugar alcohols sorbitol, mannitol, xylitol, isomaltose, and hydrogenated starch hydrolisates have calories but less than sugar. The part that does not get absorbed has an osmotic laxative effect.

Patients without celiac sprue that feel better on a gluten-free diet are probably secondary to reducing fructans in their diet.

4. High in Lactose (milk sugar)

Milk (cow, goat, sheep), yogurt especially with added lactose after fermentation, soft cheeses (Ricotta & cottage), ice cream, prepared soups and sauces, some chewing gums and anti-gas products are high in Lactulose.

5. Salicylate sensitivity

Individuals with salicylate sensitivity may have nausea, vomiting, bloating, abdominal pain and diarrhea when ingesting high-salicylate food.

Some reports indicates that up to 70% of IBS patient may be salicylate sensitive. Of these patients 20% have asthma, and 60% may have itchy rashes, headaches and/or migraines.

High-salicylates fruits and vegetables includes all dried fruits, apricot, avocado, blackberries, blueberries, boisenberry, cherries, cranberry, date, grape, guava, orange, pineapple, plum, prune, raisin, raspberry, rock melon, strawberry, tangelo and tangerine.

Vegetables very high in salicylates are peppers, radish, and tomatoes.

LOW FODMAP FOODS

Fruits: like citrus fruits, grapefruit, strawberry, blueberry, banana, grape, honeydew, cantaloupe, maple syrup and kiwi fruits all in moderation, lemon, lime, and raspberry.

Artificial Sweeteners: such as sugar, glucose, other artificial sweeteners not ending in "OL" such as sucralose (Splenda), aspartame (Equal), and saccharine (Sweet&Low).

Lactose-free dairy products, rice or almond milk, hard cheeses like cheddars, lactose-free margarine as butter substitute, brie cheese, sorbet, gelato ice cream, lactose-free yogurt. If severe lactose intolerance uses OTC Lactaid pills even with lactose-free dairy products since lactose-free products are not regulated and may not be as lactose-free as claimed. The same holds true for lactaid enzyme products (pill, capsule, drops).

Starches: such as rice, corn, potato, gluten-free cereal and bread.
Use Beano tablets (Alfa-galactosidase enzyme that breaks down complex carbohydrates) if necessary with your first bite of foods when applicable to reduce gas produced by legumes.

Gas-free soak: place 1 pound of beans in 10 cups of boiling water, boil for 2 to 3 minutes. Then cover and set aside overnight. The next day 75 to 90% of the indigestible sugars that cause gas will have dissolved into the soaking water.

Vegetables: like winter squash, lettuce, spinach, cucumber, bell pepper, green beans, tomato and eggplant.
Salicylate sensitive: fruits negligible in salicylate like pears (ripe and peeled) and lime. Vegetables with negligible salicylate include beans, cabbage, celery, split pea, lentil, iceberg lettuce, dried peas, peeled potato, almond, and peanuts.

IBS TREATMENT

E ducate about IBS and reassure in the absence of alarm signs and symptoms, and if no problem is suspected talk about the role that ethnicity (lactose intolerance) and diet (high FODMAP) has in producing IBS symptoms.

Dietary modifications (exclusion of gas producing foods and lactose avoidance), followed by low-FODMAP diet.

Adjunctive **pharmacologic** therapy:

1- **Pain** management

Anticholinergics and antispasmodics like Dicyclomine (Bently), hyoscyamine sulfate either short acting: NuLev, Levsin, Anaspaz) or long acting (Levbid)

Psychotropic agents can have neuromodulatory and analgesic properties, especially in the gut with benefits even in the absence of psychiatric co-morbidity,

> tricyclic antidepressants (TCAs) offer benefits for abdominal pain, diarrhea and depression if present, Amitriptyline start at 25 mg at bed time and increase on weekly basis, maximum dose for depression is 300 mg daily. If elderly

get EKG to make sure QTC is not more than 450 mesc. or Nortriptyline start at 10 mg at bed time, max dose for depression is 150 mg daily, Imipramine starts at 25 and Desipramine start at 10 mg.

The most common mistake is not increasing the dose by 10–25 mg every 7 days if necessary. Continue optimal dose for 6–12 months before starting to taper.

SSRIs offer benefits for IBS-D patients, begin with small dose, good in patients with depression, OCD, and anxiety. No help for pain.

Serotonin agents (agonist and antagonists depending on the type of IBS).

2- **Bloating**: anti flatulent, antispasmodics. In 75% of IBS patients bloating improves with a short course of antibiotic (Rifaximin).

3- **Diarrhea**: loperamide (OTC Imodium), diphenoxylate plus atropine (Lomotil) a Controlled V category drug, cholestyramine (Questran), and serotonin antagonist (Alosetron).

In my experience true IBS diarrhea is rarely seen. Patients are mostly females with severe diarrhea, abdominal pain and urgency of at least 3-month duration and no other cause.

Alosetron 1 mg bid (Lotronex), a 5-HT3 receptor blocker, a neuroenteric modulator, reduces colon motility and secretions. It is approved for treatment of severe diarrhea predominant IBS in females whose symptoms have lasted more than 6 months and have failed to respond to all other conventional treatment. Alosetron reduces colonic motility and secretions and may improve abdominal pain. Side effect: ischemic colitis and severe constipation. Lotronex is prescribed under restricted conditions by an enrolled prescribe program. Stop it if no better after 4 weeks.

Eluxadoline (Viberzi) 75–100 mg bid, category IV controlled drug, it is also approved for severe IBS-D patients. It has the potential for addiction and abuse. If overdose use Naloxone. Watch for side effects of acute pancreatitis, SOD in post CCY patients, and severe constipation.

Ondansetron (Zofran) anti-nausea and vomiting medication, is a 5-HT3 antagonist as wel, it may improve diarrhea but not abdominal pain in IBS.

4- **Constipation**: In the US 63 million people are suffering from chronic constipation, of those 15.3 million are assumed to be due to IBS (IBS-C), 11% have slow transit constipation, 13% are due to pelvic floor dyssynergic defecation, 5% combination of the two and the rest are considered functional.

For treatment of functional constipation increase water intake and activity, set aside a time of 30 to 60 minutes after meals, preferably after breakfast, to sit on the toilet, relax and pay attention in order to wake the gastrocolic reflex. Increase fruit and fibers.

Medications used in order of severity of constipation start with OTC **stool softeners** like docusate (Colace), followed by laxatives and saline laxatives, glycerine suppositories and enemas and then progress to stronger meds as needed.

Osmotic agents: like synthetic disaccharide Lactulose (Cephulac, Chronulac, Enulose), 25–70% Sorbitol solutions and Polyethylene glycol=PEG (Miralax) also moistens the stool. In patients with hard stool start with 17g PEG daily in 8 oz of water and increase to 34g daily if necessary (bed time).

CAUTION: Patients with kidney problems must avoid laxatives containing magnesium.

Lactulose needs 24 to 48 hours to work. Sorbitol is equally effective and less expensive. They both cause bloating and flatulence.

Starting dose with Lactulose is 10g in 20 ml water, and sorbitol 30 g (120 ml of 25% solution).

If a patient has thin and ribbon shaped stools, I will recommend a bulk forming laxative (fiber supplements), starting with a teaspoonful of raw bran or Metamucil daily, and increase to a maximum of 2 tablespoonfuls within two weeks in order to get used to the unpleasant bloating and discomfort that may result. Remember that a constipated patient with hard stools can become more constipated with added fiber supplements if they don't drink at least 8–12 tall glass of water daily.

Fiber supplements are natural or synthetic polysaccharides or cellulose derivatives that absorb water and increase fecal mass. They soften the stool and increase frequency of bowel movements.

Bulk forming laxatives in the market include psyllium (Metamucil), methyl cellulose (Citrucel), calcium polycarbophil (FiberCon), wheat dextrin (Benefiber).

Fiber gummies are soluble inulin fibers, more popular nowadays with patients, especially kids. Usual dose 2–4 pieces daily. They also increase bloating.

Apples, peaches, pears, cherries and prunes have large amount of fiber plus sorbitol.

If either a PEG solution or fiber supplements by themself don't work, a combination of Fiber and PEG works magic in majority of cases.

Treatment is ratcheted up by increasing dose and, if necessary, with additional meds like osmotic laxatives, laxative and other relatively newer but much more expensive "fancier" medications.

I'll now review briefly medicines available over the counter or by prescription. **Surfactant/emollients** are stool softeners like docusate sodium (Colace)100mg b.i.d. Stool softeners are less effective than **Stimulant laxatives:** Cascara, Ex-Lax, Senna, Correctol and

Bisacodyl (Dulcolax).

Bisacodyl 5 to 20 mg as enteric coated tablet once a day, onset of action after 6 to 12 hours when taken orally and 25 to 60 minutes when taken by suppository. Dulcolax converts into active metabolite in colon. Senna (8.6 mg Sennoid per tablet, 2 to 4 tablets daily). Senekot gummies are also available now.

Milk of Magnesia (MoM), Miralax and Lactulose are hydrating osmotic laxatives.

Dulcolax and Senokot change intestinal transport of electrolytes and increase motility. Long-term use may cause hypokalemia, salt depletion, and Protein losing enteropathy. Contrary to popular belief there is no evidence that chronic use of Dulcolax causes structural or functional impairment of the colon.

Laxatives alters the stool form and passage, when needed they produce a huge relief, but may be habit-forming for your bowel (controversial).

MOM 15–30 ml at night, fleet enema if necessary for acute relief, magnesium citrate 8–12 ounce bottle by mouth to push colon contents from above down and out.

Multiple newer medications with different mechanisms of action, variable doses and different combinations may be necessary in selective cases.

Mineral oil by mouth and mineral oil fleet enemas are lubricant laxatives, useful for patient with hard impacted stool. Leakage from anus to underpants may occur, so use a pad if necessary. Don't use in children due to risk of aspiration.

And finally newer, more expensive and fancier meds that your insurance may not approve:

Lubiprostone (Amitiza) is a locally active chloride channel activator, it increases fluid secretions into the colon, dose 8 to 24 mg daily.

Linactotide (Linzess) 74–290 mcg daily & **Plecanatide** (Trulance) 3 mg daily, they are both Guanylate Cyclades C receptor agonist. They stimulate luminal chloride secretion with passive diffusion of sodium and water with secondary effect on peristalsis.

Prucalopride (Motegrity) a serotonin 5-HT4 receptor agonist that accelerates GI transit time and may alter visceral discomfort sensation. Dose 1 mg bid.

Tegaserod (Zelnorm) 6mg bid (twice a day) for women only, commonly used TID (three times daily). It is 5HT4 agonist similar to Motegrity.

Zelnorm may cause ischemic colitis, not indicated in women 65 or older and in those with history of MI, stroke, elevated LFTs and SOD following CCY.

Methyl naltrexone 150–450 mg daily (Relistor) for Opioid-induced chronic constipation.

Management of severe constipation (obstipation and impaction) starts with glycerin or dulcolax suppositories and a fleet enema. If impacted, perform a digital disimpaction in the ER and mineral oil fleet enema plus oral magnesium citrate, provided that bowel obstruction is ruled out.

I have treated exceptions to the rule several times when patients with intractable constipation required a combination of Miralax (PEG), Metamucil, Docusate, Senna, Amitiza, Trulance and Motegrity on a daily basis.

In an institutionalized patient, in addition to routine use of Chronulac, or Cephulac plus fiber supplements, giving a fleet enema once a week and a 12 ounce bottle of magnesium citrate once every 2 weeks will help prevent recurrence of fecal impaction and visits to the ER.

In addition to fiber supplements and Miralax, for patients with significant slow transit constipation, I sometimes add Amitiza, Motegrity and Trulance to other regiments in order to increase the colonic secretion and motility required for a good bowel movement.

When dealing with dry stools constipation, Amitiza increases chloride rich fluid in the colon. Bisacodyl or Dulcolax increase both secretion and motility. Dulcolax is used less often due to fear of developing dependence. Of course, a patient with chronic constipation who needs meds for moving bowesl like Linzess, Amitiza etc. is a long-term medication user and "dependent" as well.

Finally, in some patients with severe intractable constipation appropriate **surgical procedures** like repair of rectal prolapse, rectocele, vaginocele, rectal and sigmoid prolapse, pelvic floor defects, and subtotal colectomy with Ileorectal anastomosis may be indicated and "lifesaving."

Pelvic floor physical therapy and biofeedback is helpful in patients with dyssynergic defecation. **Note** that 2/3 of patients with dyssynergic defecation also have slow transit defecation and both need to be corrected for successful outcome.

In patients with constipation and IBS symptoms of severe bloating and abdominal discomfort, a diet high in carbohydrates, fructose, lactose, gluten and High-FOMAP foods needs to be restricted, and if SIBO is present be treated.

Keep in mind the side effects of medications used for IBS like Dicyclomine for pain and TCAs for anxiety and depression, calcium channel blockers used for hypertension.

Lactulose and Sorbitol will increase symptoms of bloating and discomfort as well.

Psychotropic agents the four major classes of psychotropic agents used for IBS patients are tricyclic antidepressants (**TCAs**), selective serotonin reuptake inhibitors (**SSRIs**), serotonin-norepinephrine reuptake inhibitors (**SNRIs**) and atypical antipsychotics.

TCAs like Amitriptyline slow both small bowel and colon transit. Side effects include sedation, anticholinergics effects (constipation, tachycardia, urinary retention and dry mouth) and CNS side effects (insomnia, agitation, nightmares). Secondary amine TCAs (Desypramine, Nortriptyline) are better tolerated than tertiary amine TCAs (amitriptyline, imipramine) because of their lower anticholinergics and antihistamine properties.

SSRIs increase synaptic concentration of 5HT, and they can be used to augment the anti-anxiety effects of TCAs and reduce GI pain. They improve general well-being and depression, and unlike TCAs they don't need dose adjustment. Because of selective receptor affinity for 5HT, diarrhea may be a side effect; therefore, SSRIs may benefit patients with IBS-C. Paroxetin (Paxil) is a good choice for patients with IBS-D. Fluoxetine (Prozac) has a longer half-life and fewer withdrawal side effects, and may be selected if poor compliance is an issue. Side effects include agitation, hostility, suicidality, and diarrhea.

SNRIs (Effexor and Cymbalta) are used for IBS patients with associated OCD, ADHD, anxiety and somatic pain like fibromyalgia. Effexor can cause severe nausea in some patients.

Tenapanor (IBSRELA) a sodium/hydrogen exchange3 inhibitor enhances colon transit and stool softener, 50 mg twice daily.

COMPLEMENTARY AND ALTERNATIVE MEDICINE FOR IBS (CAM)

CAM is a diverse group of medical treatments and approaches that are not commonly considered to be a part of conventional medicine. CAM is widely used among patients with chronic medical conditions that are difficult to treat.

CAM use in IBS is highest in women with higher education and anxiety. Behavioral therapies includes cognitive behavioral therapy, mindfulness meditation, multi-component psychotherapy, psychodynamic Interpersonal therapy to identity and address difficulties in relationships, and hypnotic suggestions. CAM have been used to reduce gut unpleasant sensations.

Cognitive behavioral therapy attempts to change ways patients perceive and react to symptoms, like the use of daily diaries, and trying to increases control over symptoms.

Relaxation training uses imagery and relaxation techniques to reduce autonomic arousal and stimulate muscle relaxation.

Acupuncture may help symptoms, but studies show there's no statistically significant difference between acupuncture and sham acupuncture in relieving IBS symptoms.

Other examples of CAM used frequently in treatment of IBS are a combination of prebiotics and probiotics, acupuncture, herbal medicines, peppermint oil (reported effective), St John's Wort, and different over the counter Chinese and Japanese herbal mixtures like STW5, which is composed of bitter candytuft, chamomile flower, peppermint leaves, caraway fruit, licorice root, lemon balm leaves, celandine herbs, angelica root and milk thistle fruit.

ANTIBIOTICS

Antibiotics present a risk factor for IBS symptoms because they may reduce the useful bacteria needed for fermenting unabsorbed food, resulting in osmotic diarrhea. They are used in the treatment of SIBO (Rifaximin 550 mg tid for 2 weeks) that is seen in up to 5% of patients suffering from IBS.

Rifaximin 550 mg twice daily for 10 days can reduce abdominal discomfort, bloating and flatulence for up to 10 weeks in more than 50% of patients complaining of bloating and diarrhea even if they don't have SIBO.

PROBIOTICS (PRO-LIFE)

Probiotic is defined as a live organism that when ingested in adequate amount exert a health benefit to the host.

The most commonly used probiotics are lactic acid bacteria and non-pathogenic yeasts.

Several organisms such as Lactobacillus (L) acidophilus, L. Casei, L.GG, L. Plantarum, Bifidobacterium (B) Animalis, B. Infantis, and the probiotic cocktail VSL#3 (a mixture of 8 probiotic species of Bifidobacterium, Lactobacillus, and Streptococcus (S)) are claimed to be effective in reducing abdominal pain, flatulence, constipation and bloating.

A mixture of L bulgaricus, L. acidophilus, and S. Thermophilus, is used to ferment lactose to lactic acid, and acidic pH coagulates protein and forms yogurt. The longer yogurt stays at room temperature the more probiotic bacteria grows in it, turning lactose to lactic acid and making it taste more sour. The sour yogurt has less lactose and more probiotic bacteria.

Yogurt is said to have been brought to Turkey by Mongols millennia ago. Yogurt and wheat bread are the main staple of diet in the Middle East, and in the last 30 years it is being used more in the United States. To make it more palatable, companies are using marketing ploys like adding different fruits, honey, cereals, etc. to single use containers. That practice has additional health benefits by providing prebiotics to the live bacteria present in yogurt, and increasing the chance of bacteria in reaching the colon.

Probiotic Greek Yogurt in the US has 5 probiotics in it, including lactobacillus bulgaricus, L. acidophilus, L bifidus, L. Casei, and Streptococcus thermophilus.

Sacaromyces Bulardi (yeast) 200 to 1000 mg daily is particularly useful in reducing antibiotic associated diarrhea (C diff and post H. pylori treatment). In my experience the same or better results can be seen with probiotic yogurts.

Fortunately, the safety profile and adverse event rate of probiotics have been good; however, probiotics should be used with caution in premature infants, immunosuppressed individuals and patients with severe acute pancreatitis.

PREBIOTICS

A prebiotic is considered to be a non-digestible food ingredient that beneficially affect the host by selectively stimulating the growth and/or activity of one of a limited number of potentially health promoting bacteria in the colon, notably lactobacilli and bifidobacteria.

Prebiotic are most commonly carbohydrates from FODMAP groups.

FODMAPs are non-digestible but fermentable carbohydrates present in wheat, garlic, onions, berries, apples, pears, artichokes, asparagus, rye, bananas, soluble fiber supplements, lactulose, etc.

Short-chain FODMAP prebiotics like oligo -fructose ferments more quickly in proximal the colon. Long chain prebiotics like inulin ferments more slowly and benefits good bacteria that are present throughout the colon. Full spectrum prebiotics (oligo-fructose plus inulin) targets the entire colon. To affect a beneficiary change in gut bacteria and even change enterotype one must consume relatively large amounts of prebiotic on a daily basis. I usually recommend to all of my patients that they consume at least one serving of Activia yogurt daily, as it has billions of live probiotic bacteria and less than 100 calories. Or that they get a large container of low-fat yogurt and mix it with banana, apple, blueberry etc. (symbiotic) as a snack or replacing one meal daily.

SYMBIOTICS

Symbiotics are a combination of pre-biotics and probiotics meant to increase the survival and activity of proven probiotics in vivo. Several commercial products are available but natural yogurt mixed with fruits is the best and cheapest example.

Kefir is an excellent symbiotic originating in Russia, with consistency similar to thin yogurt, and a slightly sour taste like Ayran. It is carbonated and minimally alcoholic. It is found in the dairy section of most supermarkets. Kefir grains are fermented in milk at room temperature overnight. The bacteria in it are responsible for producing polysaccharide kefiran. Lactose in milk is consumed by fermenting bacteria to produce lactic acid, CO_2 and ethanol. Microorganisms present in Kefir includes lactobacillus kefiranofaciens, saccharomyces turicensis, lactobacillus acidophilus, bifidobacterium bifidum, streptococcus thermophilus, lactobacillus bulgaricus, and L. Helveticus, L. Lactis and yeasts like saccharomyces fragilis, saccharomyces cerevisiae, torulaspora delbrueckii and others can also ferment lactose. Kefir has all the proteins, minerals and vitamins present in milk.

IBS PHENOTYPES EXAMPLE SEEN BY ME AND RESPONDING TO THE RECOMMENDED TREATMENTS

In this segment aimed to educate providers, several patients diagnosed to have irritable bowel syndrome and on medications are presented. All are real, they were seen by me in consultation and their problems were resolved with interventions as described. The majority of patients with IBS-D will respond to reducing lactose, carbohydrates, fruits and vegetables high in FODMAP. For those suffering from IBS-C, the same dietary restrictions apply, along with a tablespoonful of Miralax (PEG) at bedtime and a cup of Bran cereal in the morning in order to relieve concomitant constipation.

A low percentage of IBS referrals to GI specialists are more complicated and require a lot more time with careful evaluation.

Obviously, to be successful in diagnosing etiology and resolving a patient's problem, the provider must be knowledgeable in differential diagnosis and aware of all of the possible conditions that can mimic IBS symptoms. They must be judicious in ordering appropriate tests and familiar with limitations in interpreting them. Providers must carefully note dietary habits, including likes and dislikes and the reason for them. This part may be readdressed in each subsequent visit if it makes sense to do so. When considering treatment they must know the mechanism of action of each drug, their potential synergistic effects, and major side effects.

Patients must never accept a simple diagnosis of IBS and leave the Drs. Office with a prescription or two for pain, diarrhea or constipation. True IBS is very rare.

The following are some examples of "complicated patients". Most had several reasons for their symptoms, and responded to prescribed treatment.

1. A young female, professional office worker, trying to keep weight down and stay in shape. Used to be constipated, has been eating salads daily, juicing different antioxidants fruits, vegetable and nuts every morning, drinks a glass of milk before going to bed to prevent osteoporosis in view of family history both mother and aunts have osteoporosis. Has been suffering from abdominal cramps and bloating interfering with sleep. Feels constipated but moves bowels a couple of times daily, never feels empty, gets urges to go but only passes gas and small stools.

   Has been diagnosed with IBS. Blood test for gluten allergy and Crohn's disease negative. Taking fiber gummies 2 daily and Dicyclomine (Bently)20 mg bid. It helps abdominal cramps but patient feels they need to take more.

   Problem:
   Constipation, inactivity, high-FODMAP diet, possible lactose intolerance, and dicyclomine use.

   Recommendation:
   Low FODMAP diet, use Lactaid milk and lactose-free dairy products. Increase activity, increase water intake, stop fiber supplements, take dicyclomine half a tablet if experiencing severe cramps. Reduce overall oral intake to maintain weight. Started on Amitiza for constipation.

2. Obese middle-aged female with type 2 diabetes, post gastric bypass 5 years ago, has been suffering from IBS for more than a year now. She weighs 245 lbs., disappointed because she has regained 60 lbs. in the last 2 years. Is using several sugarless gums daily to curb her appetite, drinking a 2-liter bottle of diet soda, and a glass of skim milk with Vitamin D for calcium supplements even though she doesn't like milk. Complaining of gas, bloating and abdominal pain. Bowel movements are irregular, has to run to toilet several times daily but passes embarrassing flatus that stinks in the office, plus small amounts of stool mixed with mucus. Recent blood test by PCP including CBC to check for anemia, thyroid function and test for Celiac disease are negative.

Problem:
Sugarless gum with Sorbitol, maldigestion and malabsorption of food (dumping) with large amount being presented to colon bacteria for fermentation. Foul smelling gas is due to high animal fat, protein and garlic use.

Recommendation:
Stop sugar-free gum and carbonated beverages. It's obvious that she need to restrict her oral intake. To reduce malodorous gas stop fried foods and garlic and use plant base protein like Soya as opposed to animal fat and proteins. The amount of lactose is the same in milk regardless of fat level; therefore, replace skim milk with lactaid added skim milk.

3. Elderly Mandarin Chinese female who had emigrated to US 3 years ago. Saw PCP for regular checkup. Complete blood counts including TFTs, urine test and screening colonoscopy were normal. The only abnormality was osteopenia on bone density test and low vitamin D level.

She was advised to take Vit D and calcium supplements. Her granddaughter went on the internet and based on gained knowledge told her to drink a lot of milk. She was drinking a gallon of regular milk every 2 days. She developed severe bloating, abdominal cramps, frequent small loose bowel movements, tenesmus and large amounts of odorless flatulence.

PCP ordered stool for culture, OVA & parasites, blood test for gluten allergy and stool for occult blood and they were negative. She was referred for consultation to tertiary medical center where I saw her.

Problem:
Lactose intolerance is almost the rule rather than exception in Chinese individuals. In China she was not drinking milk, and only occasionally eating cheese.

Recommendation:
Stop drinking milk and use over the counter calcium plus vitamin D. If constipated as a result, take OTC Docusate (Colace) 100 mg at night. Increase physical activity around the house and walk outside more often weather permitting.

4. Indian male in his late 30s, IT engineer, sponsored by a financial institution 3 years ago and moved from India to Boston. He has gained 35 lbs. since the move, mostly mid abdominal fat. His waist size has gone from 32 inches to 36. He was getting together with friends over the weekends and they had a feast of Indian foods and drank beer while watching sports and Bollywood movies. In addition to PCP, he had seen 2 specialists for bloating and abdominal pain and evaluation, including blood tests, stool for ova and parasite, colonoscopy, CT Abdomen and pelvis all normal except for fatty liver and positive blood test for Helicobacter pylori antibody. Treated with Prevpac triple therapy for 14 days, and due to persistent H pylori detected via breath test a month after finishing treatment, he was treated the second time with quadruple therapy with Pylera, that cleared HP infection. Each time his symptoms improved for a while, only to come back with a vengeance. He had a second colonoscopy and biopsy plus upper endoscopy for gastric and duodenal biopsy and it was negative. He was put on Hyoscyamine sublingual tablets to take when needed for abdominal cramps.

    He continues to have problems especially on Monday mornings. He really feels terrible with nausea, heartburn, generalized abdominal discomfort, bloating, abdominal cramps, flatus and diarrhea. He has to spend 3 hours in the bath room before he is ready to go to work. Because he is trying unsuccessfully to lose weight during the week he has been restricting his diet to a glass of skim milk with added tablespoon of honey and teaspoon of turmeric for antioxidant effect for breakfast, a cold cut sandwich with a 12 ounce can of Diet Coke for lunch. Because of bloating, he has had difficulty sleeping flat; therefore, instead of eating dinner and keeping his stomach full, he'll eat half of mid-size watermelon when he get home at 6 pm and 2 scoops of vanilla ice cream around 10pm before going to bed.

Problem:

The prevalence of lactose intolerance in the Indian population is high. Watermelon is loaded with fructose and fructans. Honey is all fructose. He overloads himself with lactose and fructose as well as fructans. His fatty liver and weight gain may be due to a high-fructose diet. Beer has gluten and alcohol increases gastric acid and gut permeability. Diet Coke adds to bloating.

Recommendation:

Stop milk, honey, ice cream and watermelon.

Go on a strict low-carb diet to lose at least 10% of body weight. Exercise 30 minutes daily. This regimen will help to lose weight, cure fatty liver and eliminate bloating, diarrhea and abdominal pain.

5. 51-year-old male referred for screening colonoscopy. While in the exam room complained about his IBS symptoms of excessive gas, bloating, 2–3 small bowel movement daily, never normal shape and mostly soft with explosive flatus and trouble at night due to abdominal dissension interfering with sleep.

Past history included metabolic syndrome, HTN, obesity, s/p MI and quadruple coronary artery bypass grafting, high cholesterol, elevated fasting blood sugar and twice normal ALT. US showed fatty liver. He has reduced alcohol to 24 cans of beer mostly on weekends and reduced smoking to less than one pack of cigarettes daily. He was advised by his cardiologist to lose weight, stop smoking and try to bring his cholesterol down by dieting. Statins for high cholesterol not given due to elevated ALT. By talking with friends and co-workers he decided to lay off red meat and animal fat, and eat mostly beans, tofu, soya for protein plus high-roughage diet, more nuts, a lot of raw garlic, and vegetables. He was juicing kale, spinach, a stick of carrot, 2 sticks of celery, one kiwi, one half of avocado, a 12 ounce glass of skim milk, one banana, a teaspoon of tumerac and a teaspoon of cinnamon powder in the morning (OMG was my reaction), dry fruits for snacks, a large Greek Salad for lunch with a 8 oz can of V8 juice, and for dinner often baked fish or chicken with broccoli and cauliflower plus one to two 6 ounce glasses of red wine. He lost 22 lbs. within 12 months. On yearly exam his FBS and ALT was normal, cholesterol was down by 20%. A routine screening colonoscopy to terminal ileum showed 2 small 5 mm adenomatous polyps that were removed.

Problem:
High-FODMAP diet

Recommendation:
Advised to stop morning juicing routine, milk, garlic, V8 juice and alcoholic beverages. Take BeanO and try to reduce **FODMAP** in beans by soaking them in water for 24 hours or use canned beans after washing them thoroughly. This patient's problem were resolved by carefully going over details of what he puts in his mouth daily and ingests. Of course, more important is having the knowledge about different ingredients that may be contributing to symptoms and to what extent they needed to be modified without "taking your eyes off the ball" of continuing beneficial diet. IBS medications, no matter which one and in what dose not only would not help him but could make his symptoms worse and start a viscous cycle of repeating blood, stool, imaging and endoscopic tests with associated anxiety, waste of time and money, QoL issues, and work absenteeism.

6. Young male mid 40s complaining of bloating, gas, cramps, and several loose bowel movements daily, was referred by PCP for evaluation of occult blood in the stool and mild iron deficiency anemia. He is a design engineer owning his own firm, in excellent health, Marathon runner, who routinely runs 10 miles daily rain or shine, working 12 hour days, not requiring much sleep, on Paleo-friendly diet, starting with smoothie in the morning, munches on mix nuts during the day, drinks more than a pot of coffee during the day, addicted to Diet Pepsi, denies alcohol and tobacco use but enjoys a couple of organic marijuana joints daily.

He takes a couple of OTC ibuprofen before running every morning.
Colonoscopy to terminal ileum and upper endoscopy with duodenal biopsy and Pill Cam studies to check small intestine for the source of occult blood were normal. Gliadin Ab IgG was positive but TTG Ab and duodenal biopsy were negative foe Celiac disease.

Problem:
Excess physical activity can cause diarrhea and occult blood in the stool possibly due to bowel ischemia and leaky gut, and over long period may cause IDA especially if diet is low in iron. Paleo diet is very high in FODMAP, he drinks large amount of coffee that may cause rapid intestinal transit. Positive Gliadin antibody may be related to leaky gut, since he had no FH of celiac sprue and HLA-DQ2 & DQ8 a prerequisite for having Celiac was negative.

Recommendation:
We discussed that majority of his symptoms could be due to his diet, and strenuous physical activity plus daily ibuprofen may have caused blood in the stool and anemia. He was advised to stay on low-gluten and low-FODMAP diet as much as he possibly can to make his symptoms tolerable,

avoid NSAIDs and take a daily multivitamin with iron for anemia and daily glutamine and zinc supplements may help leaky gut.

7. Elderly female retired health care worker presented with increasing IBS symptoms of severe watery diarrhea, abdominal cramps of several years duration that is getting worse in the last couple of years in spite of taking recommended: Colestipol (Cholestyramine) two tablets twice daily (4 G), Peptobismul 15 ml at bed time, Metamucil one tablespoonful twice daily and Imodium AD 2 mg tablet twice a day. She is S/p multiple SBO due to intraabdominal adhesions, treated with hospitalization and intestinal decomposition by nasogastric tube twice, and once required laparoscopic surgery for release of adhesion. She was told that her abdomen was matted with adhesions. S/p Hystrectomy for uterine fibromyoma in her 40s and removal of gallbladder for acute cholecystitis 5 years ago. She has been taking Naprosyn 500 mg bid for severe bilateral osteoarthritis in her knees x 4 years, causing gastric ulcer bleed for several months following start of taking it, requiring hospitalization, endoscopic dual therapy and 2 units blood transfusion, gastric biopsy showed *helicobacter pylori* infection of stomach with chronic gastritis. H.pylori was eradicated and confirmed at the time by both stool for H pylori Ag and breath test.

Upon hospital discharge she was advised to take Lansoprazole 30 mg twice daily as long as she takes Naprosyn twice a day to prevent recurrence of ulcer.
After obtaining history and with a negative abdominal exam Colonoscopy and biopsy was done.

Problem:
Severe episodes of watery diarrhea, including nocturnal, and occasional fecal incontinence. This was diagnosed to

be secondary to post cholecystectomy bile acid-induced diarrhea, treated with Cholestyramine, a bile acid binding resin and she improved.

She was incapacitated due to arthritis in knees and had refused surgery. She had difficulty ambulating and was using a cane. Daily high-dose Naprosyn was helpful and necessary, but it caused bleeding ulcer in combination with H pylori infection of stomach. High-dose Lansoprazole was added daily in order to prevent recurrence of ulcer while continuing Naproxyn.

She was prone to getting SBO due to intraperitoneal adhesions and has been advised by her surgeon to stay on low-roughage soft diet to prevent bowel obstruction.

This patient appeared to be suffering from bile acid-induced diarrhea secondary to CCY, SIBO due to adhesion-induced SB strictures and stagnation, and possible microscopic colitis secondary to any or all of the following meds; Naprosyn, lansoprazole and peptobismul use.

Recommendation:
Lactulose breath test was positive for SIBO showing >20ppm Hydrogen.

Colonoscopy and biopsy showed microscopic and collagenous colitis.

She was treated with 2 weeks course of Rifaximin followed by budesonide (Entecort) 9 mg daily. On the long-term she requires twice a year antibiotic for severe bloating heralding recurrent SIBO, and able to tolerate coming off maintenance budesonide 3 mg daily for 6–8 weeks. lansoprazole was switched to pantoprazole 40 mg bid and peptobismul was stopped.

She continues with Colestipol tablets for bile acid diarrhea and takes Imodium prior to going for a ride or Doctors appointment.

She requires occasional short course of antibiotics for SIBO and Budesonide for recurring microscopic colitis.

8. Middle-aged female with several years of occasional mid abdominal pain, cramp, urgency and diarrhea that is getting worse and takes up to 24 hours for discomfort to clear. Evaluation including appropriate blood and stool tests, colonoscopy, upper endoscopy with SB biopsy has been negative. On further questioning she mentioned that going out to dinner was a pleasure before, but now dines out twice weekly and some nights are interrupted by cramps, severe bloating, abdominal pain and diarrhea and she has to get home because of extreme gas, bloating, pain and the urge that if not relieved may lead to a loss of bowel control.

Problem:
It appeared that she may be suffering from some kind of food allergy. She was advised to keep a chart of restaurants that she frequents and the type of food that she eats before becoming symptomatic.
Finally, she determined that garlic is the ingredient that is causing symptoms. Avoiding garlic has eliminated her symptoms. She was telling me that unfortunately most food, in most restaurants has added garlic and has had to stop going out to dinner. She even once had a Bagel at *Finagle a Bagel* café and the bread knife cutting her bagel has been used to cut a bagel with garlic just before hers, and she had similar but less severe symptoms.

Recommendation:
Food sensitivity and allergy is becoming a more frequent cause of IBS symptoms. Pattern of presentation should alert physician to help patient pinpoint offending food. Occasionally patient needs to see a allergist to find the allergen and desensitize if possible.
Several years later she developed dysphagia to solids due to "feline esophagus" by Barium swallow since she refused endoscopy and biopsy, and also allergy to chicken and

eggplant with similar symptoms. She avoids these foods and refuses any evaluation or treatment.

9. Middle-aged male presented with increasing abdominal bloating, cramps, excess foul-smelling gas "like a rat died inside me," 3–4 soft mushy stools. He was a chef at a busy resturant and running to the BR frequently for him plus excess foul-smelling gas bothered coworkers in a contained kitchen space and they begged him to see a Doctor.

Reviewing his diet carefully he stated that he loves the smell of freshly baked bread and can live on that if he has to, he eats mostly freshly baked bread with garlic in olive oil throughout the day when he feels hungry, and a large bowl of plain pasta prepared with garlic and butter at night. However, his breakfast is complete and included 6 strips of bacon with 4 fried eggs, a stack of pancakes with butter and maple syrup, a tall glass of orange juice and 2 cups of coffee with cream. He'll drink 3 shots of double espresso coffee during the day and 6 bottles of Corona beer at night when busy cooking. He used to drink heavily and has been hospitalized twice when younger for acute pancreatitis secondary to alcohol and on his last admission he was scared when he was told that in addition to acute pancreatitis he also has alcoholic hepatitis and if he doesn't stop drinking alcohol he will die from liver cirrhosis. He stopped drinking cold turkey for 5 years. drinking restarted with toasting a glass of champagne at his brother's wedding. He was the Best man and felt like one drink won't harm, even though he knew better. Now he drinks only beer and no hard liquor and attends AA meetings anytime he gets a chance. He used to smoke cigarettes 2 ppd for at least 20 years. He stopped smoking when in prison for 3 month and is back to vaping tobacco now.

Evaluations revealed only fatty liver by ultrasound and low pancreatic elastase in the stool.

Problem:

Risk factors for Chronic pancreatitis and pancreatic insufficiency include alcohol abuse, cigarettes smoking and history of acute pancreatitis twice.

On high FODMAP, high gluten (bread, pasta, beer, garlic) high-fat (olive oil, butter, bacon,) diet, supplemented with excess coffee (rapid intestinal transit) and beer.

Foul smelling flatus: egg, garlic and excess fat.

Maldigestion: chronic pancreatitis.

Recommendation:

He was advised to stop bread with olive oil and garlic during the day, cut back in bacon and eggs in the morning, and have pasta with marinara sauce instead of butter and garlic and reduce coffee drinking.

Low pancreatic elastase in the stool indicated pancreatic insufficiency and he was started on Creon 36000 to take 2 with breakfast and 2 with dinner to begin with.

10. Middle-age patent attorney with long standing Crohn's colitis off Humira for couple of years because Colitis has been under control for the last 3 years. He was suffering from Episodes of severe mid abdominal pain and cramps lasting from few minutes to hours and occasionally with vomiting, but always nausea, bloating followed by explosive diarrhea. Colonoscopy showed mild peri-appendiceal and distal rectal erythema. Terminal ileum endoscopy and biopsy negative for Crohn's. CRP and stool calprotectin and occult blood was negative. He was being treated for anxiety and IBS at this point with lorazepam, donnatal extentab twice daily and levsin SL when necessary for pain. Because of recurring episodes of transient severe mid abdominal pain, he underwent small bowel camera study/pill cam, to check for evidence of segmental Crohn's in the Small intestine. Possibility of camera getting stuck

requiring surgery if stricture is present due to Crohn's discussed and he consented to proceed. Alternatives MRE & CTE evaluating small intestine by MRI or CT scan was not a choice. He is claustrophobic unwilling to have MRE, and has had multiple CT abdomen and pelvis before and due to low sperm count he was trying to avoid CT unless absolutely necessary.

When reviewing SB Camera pictures, I could not believe my eyes when I saw multiple ascaris worms residing in mid small bowel region. I called him to inform him about this finding, He said that in the last 3 years and since he moved to a new international law firm in Boston he has been traveling for business to the Middle East, India and Africa several times.

Problem:
This patient is very well informed about Crohn's, staying on lactose-free, low residue bland diet, colitis is in remission as shown by annual colonoscopy. Previously no evidence of SB Crohn's. Yet episodes of pain, twice prompting ER visit with negative blood tests and pancreatic enzymes studies. Kub / plain x ray of abdomen reported nonspecific SB gas pattern, may be ileus. He improves just before reaching ER or while there and is discharged with Dx of IBS.
Knowing this patient for years, I could not buy IBS as a diagnosis, prompting the Pill Cam study.
He thought that the source of parasite infestation may have been India. We discussed that this may have brought his Crohn's under control.

Recommendation:
Mebendazole 100 mg bid x 3 days, with 500 mg repeat in 3 weeks. He noticed passage of several worms both times.

He has been off Humira and has had no problem with Crohn's colitis or IBS symptoms as long as he is careful with his diet.

11. Retired RN, with 2 years of watery diarrhea, abdominal cramps and weight loss. 2 hospital admissions within 6 months for dehydration and low potassium. Comprehensive evaluation of blood, stools including PCR negative, CT abdomen and pelvis, SB biopsy, colonoscopy with biopsy, normal, urine 5HIAA pancreatic hormone VIP known to cause watery diarrhea and hypokalemia negative. Even stool check for factitious laxatives abuse was negative. In view of negative work up and continuing symptoms eluxadoline (Viberzi) was added to 8 mg Imodium and 4 diphenoxylate (lomotil) daily. Empiric Trial of budesonide (entecort) for possible AIE and Mic Colitis in spite of negative biopsies not effective either. She continued with watery diarrhea and weight loss. Sandostatin SC injection twice daily offered some benefits in slowing down diarrhea. Octreotide whole body scan revealed slight uptake in RUL of lung. Chest x-ray showed 4 cm mass RUL. Biopsy showed small cell lung cancer. RU Lobectomy resolved diarrhea.

Problem:
I saw this patient with diagnosis of severe watery diarrhea in a female with IBS. During her previous hospital admission comprehensive evaluations has ruled out bacterial, viral, organic and structural abnormalities and IBS remained diagnosis of exclusion. She was put on empiric budesonide therapy at a tertiary center without effect.
After reviewing her medical records as it related to diarrhea, I was impressed by persistent watery diarrhea and 2 admissions because of low potassium, a classic presentation for VIPoma, a pancreatic endocrine tumor. Repeat serum VIP level and special pancreas CT scan was negative. Because

diarrhea slowed down with Sandostatin, I proceeded with ordering whole body Octreotide scan. Minimal uptake in RUL of lungs was seen. To my surprise no CXR has been done in the last 10 years. A Chest X-ray was done and the rest is history. Mary is doing well, healthy, has regained her weight and has no more diarrhea since the lung cancer was removed.

Recommendation:
Mary was referred to thoracic surgery and Oncology. Biopsy showed lung cancer, no evidence of metastasis. Removal of the lung lobe containing mass resolved diarrhea. The tumor has been secreting VIP hormone. Small cell Lung cancer is known to cause paraneoplastic syndrome and this case was a very rare form of such manifestations.

She has been complaining of cough, occasionally associated with large amount of fluid expectoration; however, this was attributed to her cigarette smoking history and chronic bronchitis and conveniently ignored. To everyone's surprise she never had a Chest X-ray during hospital admissions. Chest X-ray used to be a necessary routine prior to admission but not anymore.

12. Elderly female with episodes of severe diarrhea, preceded by intense lower abdominal cramp and occasional incontinence. Stools are watery, explosive and yellowish in color. She had gall bladder surgery many years ago. On dicyclomine (Bently) 20 mg. twice daily for years now. She was told by previous gastroenterologist that her diarrhea is related to her gall bladder removal and free-flowing bile acts like a laxative. She was Put on Colestipol 1g tablets to take 2 tablets twice daily, after couple of years she cut it back to 2 tablets daily and eventually stopped it because they were too big to swallow and she claimed that it was not helping anyway. She takes up to 4 lomotil (diphenoxylate) daily and has difficulty getting refill from her PCP.

Problem:
Bile acid-induced diarrhea is seen in 10% of patients after CCY and persist in up to 3% of patients for life.

Recommendation:
She was started on Metamucil 15 G daily to solidify her stools and cholestyramine powder (Questran)4 gram twice daily. She was told to dissolve each packet in 8 ounce of orange juice and take it after lunch and dinner. She was on thyroid hormone in the morning. Cholestyramine powder needs to be taken within 4 hours of other medications, since it may bind them and reduce effective level in the blood. Diarrhea stopped and no more need for Lomotil.
She was told to take an Imodium tablet before going out for reassurance. She was able to reduce her Questran dose to 4 G daily after 6 months.
Cholestyramine powders is easier to take in higher dose and in my opinion more effective than the large Colestid pills.

13. Elderly female with 8 years of watery diarrhea several times a day and at night, diaper dependent to cover up for diarrheal incontinence. On 2-liter nasal oxygen at home for dyspnea secondary to COPD and CHF. On omeprazole 20 mg daily since her second heart surgery that she did not know the indication for it and nobody has tried to figure it out and take her off it if not necessary, 2 blood thinners, Coumadin and Plavix (Clopidogrel) for Atrial Fibrillation, that has recurred post ablation, s/p Remote CVA with minimal residual, mechanical aortic valve replacement, mitral valve repaire and triple vessel CABG. She has been evaluated for chronic diarrhea many times and was on fiber supplement, diphenoxylate and will consume 4 DTO drops before going for a ride or to Drs office.

She has never had a colonoscopy due to her advanced age of 89, comorbid conditions and the fact that she could not come off anticoagulation and will need several days of hospital admission with heparin bridge and prep for colonoscopy.

Problem:
Pattern of diarrhea, age, sex, and medications that mentioned are compatible with microscopic/ collagenous colitis.

Recommendation:
I discussed with the patient and her daughter that she most likely has microscopic colitis. She said previous consultant had guessed the same. Furthermore, I suggested that due to this interfering with her QoL even more than COPD and heart-related issues, and in the absence of contraindications, consider therapeutic trial of oral Budesonide (Entecort) 3 mg tablet, 9 mg in the morning after breakfast. They both agreed. My office received multiple calls from thankful patient and her daughter. According to her "I can walk on water." After 2 years she is down to 3 mg

budesonide tablet every other day with 1–3 bowl movements daily.

14. Patient with Ehlers Donlos syndrome and controlled HIV on maintenance treatment. IBS symptoms evaluated and was found to have lactose intolerance, and SIBO treated with 14 days of Rifaximin 550 mg three times daily and cleared. In spite of strict lactose-free diet continues to have abdominal discomfort, diarrhea and bloating with multiple foods. He read it on the internet that Ehlers Donlos patients suffer from leaky gut and was taking glutamine and zinc supplements to treat it. He presented to tertiary center asking for lactulose-mannitol urine and blood tests to determine if he has leaky gut and if so how serious it is.

I informed him that unfortunately we are not equipped to do LM urine test, that not everyone accepts leaky gut as an entity and he should continue with his supplements and avoid NSAIDs, and to have Immunoglobulin level to r/o CVID. He left GI clinic disappointed. He was a PhD in chemistry and has read everything there is to know about IBS and every possible test done at least twice. It is difficult to satisfy a patient that is "more knowledgeable" than the Doctor.

15. Middle-aged male, overweight presented because of early satiety, nausea, post prandial bloating, increased flatulence, abdominal discomfort and irregular bowel habits. He has type 2 diabetes mellitus, requiring metformin and 3 months ago started on weekly Trulicity (GLP-1 receptor agonist) injections. Past history of intraabdominal lymphoma treated by chemotherapy and radiation. A year ago, evaluated for IBS symptoms and was found to have SIBO. SB X-Ray was normal. Treated with 14 days of Rifaximin and markedly improved; however, symptoms returned 6 month ago and it is becoming intolerable now.

Problem:
Diabetes can cause gastroparesis due to visceral neuropathy. In addition dulaglutide (Trulicity and Ozempic) works by inducing gastroparesis in order to reduce appetite by inducing early satiety and oral intake, helping to lose weight in overweight diabetics. Nausea, post-prandial bloating and early satiety is most likely caused or worsened by Trulicity. Metformin also interfere with carbohydrate absorption and can result in bloating, gas and diarrhea. Radiation can cause stricture, slow intestinal transit and leaky gut. SIBO can cause leaky gut and IBS symptoms as well.

Recommendation:
Patient was advised to check with his PCP to stop metformin and Trulicity and use one of many alternative medications to control blood sugar.
He is a "set up" to have recurring and chronic SIBO because of radiation to intestines and visceral neuropathy from diabetes.
Hydrogen breath test with lactulose was positive for both Hydrogen and Methane. He was started on low-FOD-MAP diet, Rifaximin 550 mg tid x 2 weeks and added Neomycin 500 mg bid x 2 weeks because of additional

methane-producing bacteria in small intestine. He was advised that he may need to stay on long-term low-dose antibiotic daily or one week a month if and when recurrent SIBO symptoms.

16. Middle-aged male, in his late 30s, suffering years of IBS symptoms, and extensive evaluation has revealed lactose intolerance, staying off milk and ice cream, on multiple meds including limbitrol 10–25 bid (librium +amitriptyline) to control symptoms of cramps, irregular bowel movements with diarrhea predominance, and bloating.

When seen I went over his diet and nothing noteworthy to explain his symptoms and assumed he has true IBS and refilled Limbitrol prescription. During required second visit 12 months later to refill limbitrol, I asked again about his diet and possible hidden source of lactose. It was then that he "shamefully" admitted that he is a "chocoholic" and eats a pound of *Fanny Farmers* chocolate daily.

Problem:
Chocolate and caramel contain 30–40-gram fructose per 100 gram and butter. By enjoying a lbs. of chocolate daily, he was overloading his small intestinal capacity for fructose absorption, escaping large amount to colon to be fermented and produce his symptoms.

Recommendation:
I told him that chocolate is causing his symptoms, and advised to get off chocolate and taper Limbitrol. He was not willing to give up either and transferred his care to my associates.

17. Middle-aged female s/p ileitis with resection of Terminal ileum more than a decade ago for T.I Crohn's disease, was referred by surgeon for colonoscopy evaluation prior to neo-terminal ileum resection for recurrent Crohn's disease stricture not responding to medications and requiring several hospital admissions for abdominal pain, vomiting and SBO. She was also complaining about several liquid bowel movements daily, severe bloating and cramps. She was on iron tablet daily, B12 shots monthly, Pentasa full dose, Naprosyn 500 mg twice daily for hip pain, Lomotil four times daily and Demerol 50 mg every 6 hours for incapacitating bilateral hip pain and low-dose prednisone for secondary adrenal insufficiency. Labs were normal including CRP and Sedimentation rate. She had been hospitalized on multiple occasions because of SBO, relived by I.V. Fluids, NG suction and bowel rest, each lasting from 12–36 hours. Imaging including Plain abdominal X ray, CT and SB X ray have shown stricture at the ileocolic anastomosis. The reason for original T.I resection was bilateral aseptic necrosis of femoral heads due to long-term prednisone, used to treat Crohn's exacerbations (before biologic era). She had refused surgery for bilateral hip replacement.

On physical exam abdomen was bloated with hyperactive bowel sounds and mild RLQ tenderness.
Colonoscopy was normal except for a tight inflammatory stricture of the ileo-colic anastomosis. After ballon dilatation I was able to enter ileum using pediatric colonoscope. The was no evidence of Crohn's, however 20 cm in, there was a circumferential stricture and about 15 cm proximal to that another stricture typical of NSAID-induced stricture. This stricture did not allow passage of scope.

Problem:
Recurring SBO due to undigested materials like mushrooms, potato and tomato skin as well as not well chewed

corn, grapes, etc. getting stuck at the ileocolic stricture site and causing bowel obstruction requiring time to get fermented and allow peristalsis to do its job carrying it to the colon, and SIBO due to both strictures and narcotics slowing peristalsis.

Diarrhea, severe bloating and abdominal discomfort was related to severe SIBO as documented by Lactulose breath test, bile acid malabsorption secondary to incomplete absorption in the ileum and bile acid changes by by SIBO bacteria and resection of TI, B12 and Iron deficiency due to TI resection, and malnutrition respectively.

Recommendation:
Surgery was canceled much to the surgeon's disappointment. She was put on a low-residue diet and advised to go on clear liquids as soon as she feels SBO is going to start. Use lactaid milk and calcium plus vit D supplements. High-dose Pentasa (5 ASA, specific for small intestine) that was being used to treat Crohn's was stopped, she was started on Rifaximin 550 mg tid x 2 weeks followed by 550 mg daily and cholestyramine 4 G daily. She was encouraged to have hip replacement and in between she was started on liquid Naprosyn.

She has not been admitted to the hospital for SBO for several years.

Presently she is off Naprosyn, Pentasa, and narcotics. She required balloon dilatation of ileocolic anastomoses tight stricture a couple of more times within the first 2 years when she would take occasional Naproxen tablets.

18. Vry nice and polite middle-aged male, passive aggressive, executive in excellent health was referred for evaluation of several years of severe abdominal cramps, borborygmia (very noisy stomach) and explosive large volume watery diarrhea when in stressful situations like meeting for new big sales, meeting with company executives, etc. He would take 2 Lomotil tablet before anticipated problem. He thought that it helps a bit but then it constipates him for days. He was worried that one of these times he may lose control of his bowel, and always makes sure that a toilet is nearby his meeting place. He had no problem during normal daily life.

He has been evaluated before by blood tests, colonoscopy, etc. by competent gastroenterologist and upon reviewing copy of his medical record at his disposal, I could not think of any other indicated test to order.

Problem:

I felt that this is one of the rare occasions that I see a true IBS and symptoms are most likely neuro-hormonal and due to conditional excess Serotonin secretion in the intestinal tract. Mast cell Activation syndrome was not considered due to lack of urticaria and flushing that occurs with abdominal cramp and watery mucusy diarrhea when upset. He was advised to take a 1 mg Alosetron (Lotronex) tablet 30–60 minutes just before going to meetings plus one Imodium 2mg tablet.

Alosetron selectively blocks 5-HT3 (serotonin) receptors, which are extensively distributed on enteric motor neurons and in peripheral afferent and central locations such as vomiting center. These receptors modulate visceral pain, colonic transit and gastrointestinal secretions. It decreases brain activity of central autonomic network.

Alosetron is more efficacious in women with IBS-D.

His problem has resolved and now, "just to be on the safe side" he take half of Lotronex tablet when necessary.

19. A middle-age retired radiologist had moved from Boston suburbs to the upper Cape Cod area 3 years ago. He has been healthy all his life, physically active playing golf a couple of days per week, works in his garden and swims daily laps. However, in the last couple of years is not himself. He feels bloated all the times no matter what he eats, he has stopped his favorite snack of cheese and red wine in the evening because he has been having cramps, bloating and several diarrhea bowel movements with explosive gas, and his spouse added intolerable foul-smelling gas to the list. The only change in his diet was eating a lot fresher sea food and when stopped eating it for couple of weeks it did not make any difference. Saw a gastroenterologist, Colonoscopy, stool for occult blood, CRP, and TTG Ab to check for Celiac was negative. He was put on low-FOD-MAP diet, Gas-x, BeanO when necessary and Dicyclomine 20 mg every morning with partial improvement.

Upon going over his history I asked him if he traveled to foreign countries, hunting, drinking well water, he mentioned that he has a private well water at home that he uses for his garden and sometimes when attending his garden and feels thirsty he drinks couple of mouthful from it "Bingo," I said after hearing that. I ordered stool for O&P plus Giardia and cryptosporidium antigen. To my pleasant surprise stool for Giardia Ag was positive. Serum IgA level ordered subsequently was normal. He responded favorably to treatment of Giardiasis.

20. A very busy car dealership manager in his early 40s was referred for evaluation of frequent loose mucusy bowel movements and LLQ discomfort before going to work in the mornings, that sometimes delays starting daily sales meeting.

On exam LLQ was mildly tender. Evaluations including blood tests, TSH, and breath tests for lactose malabsorption was negative. His diet consisted mostly of sandwich meats, steak and potatoes. He did not like fruits and vegetables. Colonoscopy showed diffuse diverticulosis from proximal rectum to the cecum, marked circular muscle hypertrophy specially in sigmoid colon and active spastic peristaltic type of activity requiring glucagon to calm his colon down during colonoscopy.

Diagnosis of Spastic Colon was made. He was put on a cup of full bran cereal in the morning with several glasses of water a day, told to eat more fruits and vegetables, plus Dicyclomine 20 mg four times daily. He has remained on the same regimen for more than 2 decades. He loves fruits and vegetables now. He was advised to see a psychiatrist for management of anxiety and depression.

21. Twenty-six year old female, dental student who recently moved from NYC to Boston was seen in the clinic with several years of IBS, manifested specially by post prandial diarrhea and urgency, worse with fried foods and up to 5 soft, bile colored watery stools daily. Denied pain or bloating. She has been evaluated extensively twice since childhood and nothing has been found. Lomotil helps prevent urgency and frequency but cause bloating that becomes intolerable during monthly menstrual periods.

Problem:
Presentation suggested Bile Acid (BA)-induced diarrhea. Since there was no history of Crohn's disease or gallbladder surgery, primary BA-induced IBS-D was considered. This could be a genetic issue related to BA overproduction by the liver or poor absorption by terminal ileum.

Recommendation:
Instead of refilling the Lomotil prescription only, I discussed the possibility of BA-induced diarrhea and gave her a choice of empirical treatment to see if it works. She enthusiastically accepted my offer. I then went over treatment of trying Cholestyramine powder that binds the excess bile and carries it out or trying a more novel approach of taking Obethicolic acid (OCALIVA) tablets that reduces BA production by the liver.

Her insurance denied coverage for OCALIVA tablet, she was then put on Colestipol 2G twice daily with marked improvement in stool urgency, frequency and shape within 2 weeks' time.

22. Highly educated African-American female in her early 40s, well known to me with GERD on Cimetidine 400 mg BID, H Pylori gastritis s/p treatment with eradication, IBS due to lactose intolerance on lactose-free diet and lactaid supplements prn, seen in the office for yearly follow up visit. On passing mentioned that her IBS has been getting worse with lower abdominal discomfort, bloating and 2–3 loose bowel movements daily, in spite of watching her lactose intake and even trying gluten-free diet. On exam there was very mild RLQ tenderness but it was around her monthly menstrual period time. On reviewing her medication list, I noticed a couple of eye drops one being steroids and when asked for how long and why is she taking them, she laughed and said she had been diagnosed with Iritis/uveitis few month ago and forgot to tell you about it. Needless to say, I scheduled her for colonoscopy and she was found to have mild terminal ileitis with multiple aphtus ulcers and positive biopsy for Crohn's. She was put on adalimumab injection. Both iritis and "IBS" symptoms resolved within a few month.

This case would have been mistreated as IBS and lead to restricting her diet perhaps severely, or added new antispasmodic if I would not have looked at her medication list and if my office staff had not updated her med list on the computer.

Made in United States
North Haven, CT
20 August 2023

40551177R00068